LABORATORY ACTIVITIES FOR LIFE SPAN MOTOR DEVELOPMENT

Kathleen M. Haywood, PhD
University of Missouri-St. Louis

Human Kinetics Books
Champaign, Illinois

Senior Editor: Gwen Steigelman, PhD
Production Director: Ernie Noa
Projects Manager: Lezli Harris
Assistant Editor: Julie Anderson
Copy Editor: Molly Bentsen
Proofreader: Wendy Petersen
Typesetter: Sandra Meier
Text Design: Keith Blomberg
Text Layout: Jane Axtell
Photographs By: Kathleen M. Haywood
Printed By: Versa Press

ISBN: 0-87322-134-6

Printed in the United States of America

10   9   8   7   6   5   4   3

Human Kinetics Books
A Division of Human Kinetics Publishers, Inc.
Box 5076, Champaign, IL 61825-5076
1-800-747-4457

Canada Office:
Human Kinetics Publishers, Inc.
P.O. Box 2503, Windsor, ON N8Y 4S2
1-800-465-7301 (in Canada only)

Europe Office:
Human Kinetics Publishers (Europe) Ltd.
P.O. Box IW14
Leeds LS16 6TR
England
0532-781708

ACKNOWLEDGMENTS

Planning these laboratory activities was an enjoyable task, in part because many people lent their talents to the effort. Catherine Lewis, a physical education teacher at Andrews Academy in St. Louis County, Missouri, read the laboratory exercises and made valuable suggestions. Many helpful suggestions on the observation guides in Part II were made by Stephen Langendorfer of Kent State University in Ohio. He generated a set of guides independently to help assure that no major point was left out. Joyce Espiritu of Parkway School District in St. Louis County, Missouri, made available the data for laboratories in Parts IV and V. Matthew, Christina, and Laura Haywood, and Kenneth and Jennifer Sweeney were cooperative in performing for the pictures. Many of the charts and tables were typed and retyped by Ann Wagner, who also did the word processing. Thanks again to all of these friends.

Contents

PREFACE

Motor development is an expanding area of study. Our knowledge of age-related changes in skill performance over the life span is increasing by leaps and bounds. There is little doubt that we primarily gain this knowledge through the written word. Yet often the concepts and ideas that remain with us the longest are gained by action and more extensive involvement than merely "reading about."

These laboratory activities were generated to provide such opportunity for more extensive involvement in basic motor development concepts and issues. After the topic is introduced in each laboratory exercise, you gather your own data, analyze your results, and compare them to the existing body of knowledge. The process is one of exploration. Often knowledge "self-discovered" is appreciated and comprehended beyond information merely presented to us.

The observation and assessment of motor performance requires training and practice, and these laboratory activities also provide experience and practice in assessing various aspects of physical growth and motor development. Many students find systematic assessment to be their most frequent application of this body of knowledge as they begin teaching careers. The materials and charts in the laboratories on assessing basic motor skills are designed to be useful beyond this initial experience.

A final benefit of laboratory activities is the opportunity for future teachers to practice bridging the gap between "knowing about" motor development and planning meaningful, appropriate learning experiences based on their knowledge. Several laboratories provide an opportunity to practice this important aspect of instruction.

Perhaps most importantly, these laboratory experiences are meant to be enjoyable, challenging ways to deepen your knowledge and appreciation of this fascinating area of study.

Kathleen M. Haywood

INTRODUCTION

This manual is divided into five parts that group the laboratory activities on related topics. There is at least one activity related to every chapter of the textbook (except the overview), however, the number of laboratories per chapter is not equal. There are several reasons for this. First, some areas of study lend themselves to "hands-on" activities while others do not. Second, future teachers benefit more from extensive practice and experience on those assessments they are more likely to conduct in educational settings. Third, other courses in this area of study likely will provide additional experiences related to some of the laboratory activities included here.

Each laboratory activity begins with an introduction that relates the activity to material covered in the textbook, *Life Span Motor Development*. One or more objectives state the goal(s) in completing the exercise. You will conduct some laboratory activities on your own. Others will be done during class or laboratory time in your assigned campus facility, and still others will be completed in clinical settings. Your instructor may arrange for you to visit a particular school or program or may ask you to locate participants for these laboratory exercises yourself. Most of the laboratory activity can be conducted in less than an hour. You will then need 15 to 20 minutes to answer the discussion questions at the end of each laboratory.

You will gain the most from your laboratory experiences if you prepare ahead of time. Each laboratory activity lists the section(s) of your textbook related to the laboratory topic. Be thoroughly familiar with this material. You also should read the entire laboratory assignment, including the discussion questions, before starting the activities. This will enable you to plan your time effectively and to attend to the important topics identified by the discussion questions as you conduct your activities.

In some laboratories you will take measurements and record them on a data sheet provided in this book. Be sure to make measurements precisely and carefully. Record numbers accurately. A common source of error occurs by reversing digits—intending to write "65" but recording "56"—so guard against this mistake. Accurate data will allow more meaningful comparisons between your results and the body of knowledge in motor development.

You will be asked to graph the results of your observations or calculations in several laboratory exercises. Usually the graph is provided but you label the axes. Determine the range in which your numerical results fall and then label the axis by distributing the range in equal increments (units of measure) over the length of the axis. For example, if your scores range from 6 to 37, label the axis from 5 to 40 using as much of the width or height of the graph as possible.

The discussion questions are provided to stimulate a deepening and broadening of your knowledge of motor development, as well as to reinforce basic concepts. Review the relevant material in your textbook and relate this material to your laboratory findings as you respond to the questions; avoid brief "yes" or "no" answers. This will be very important if your findings are not what you expected following your initial reading of the textbook. You should explain why your findings differ from the expected. You may be able to identify one or more factors that make the critical difference in your data. Whenever possible use numerical results from your measurements or calculations to support your answers.

PART

I

Physical Growth and Maturation

The assessment of growth and maturation is helpful in tempering our expectations for skill performance in children. Often children who are physiologically mature relative to their chronological age perform above average in sport and other physical activities. Children who are smaller in physical stature and less mature for their chronological age may perform below average when they are young but develop into relatively better-skilled performers at an older age. A knowledge of realistic expectations can help keep children from becoming discouraged if they are simply maturing at a slower rate than others.

As discussed in your textbook, it is difficult to assess maturation directly. Often the extent or rate of growth is measured, and maturation is implied from that measurement. The three laboratory activities in Part I are designed to help you to distinguish between assessing growth and assessing maturation, to provide practice in taking growth measurements, and to enable you to begin making implications about maturation from growth measurements.

1

Assessing Skeletal Maturation

One of the direct measures of physiologic maturation is hand and wrist X rays. Although there often are limitations on how readily these can be obtained, being familiar with the process in which an individual's X ray is compared to a standard X ray teaches us the difference between physiologic maturation and chronological age. Children of a given age can vary widely in physiologic maturation; hence, it is important to temper your expectations of children's physical performance with knowledge of their physiologic maturation.

Objective
• To become familiar with the assessment of physiologic maturation through hand and wrist X rays by comparing examples of simulated X rays.

Format
Independent work

Textbook Readings
"Skeletal Age" on pages 30-32 and "Skeletal Growth" on pages 48-52

Procedure
1. Study the simulated X ray of the hand and wrist of a six-year-old girl in Figure 1.1. Note the number of wrist bones (carpals) ossified, the extent of their ossification, and the extent of ossification at the epiphyseal growth plates located at the ends of the long bones of the hand (metacarpals and phalanges) and forearm (radius and ulna). This simulated X ray is the standard for a girl 6.0 years old.

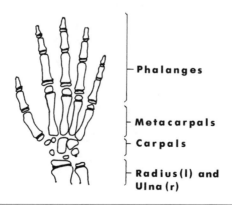

Phalanges

Metacarpals

Carpals

Radius (l) and Ulna (r)

Figure 1.1

2. Now study the simulated X ray in Figure 1.2 for the same features listed above. Complete the Analysis Table by filling in the column for Figure 1.2. Do the same for the simulated X ray in Figure 1.3, then answer the discussion questions.

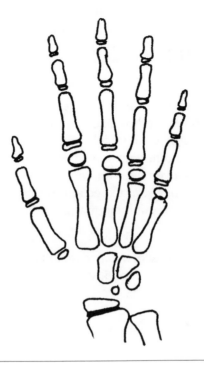

Figure 1.2

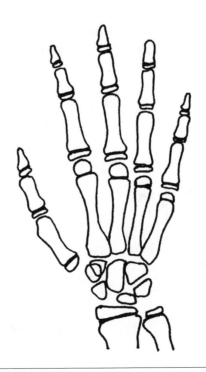

Figure 1.3

Name _____ Section _____ Date _____

LABORATORY 1: ASSESSING SKELETAL MATURATION
Analysis Table

Directions: Enter "M" (More) if the number of ossification centers or the extent of ossification is more than the standard, "L" (Less) if it is less, or "S" (Same) if it is the same.

Criteria	Figure 1.2	Figure 1.3
Number of wrist bone (carpals) ossified		
Growth plate at distal end of radius		
Growth plate at distal end of ulna		
Growth plates of the metacarpals		
Growth plates of the phalanges		

Discussion Questions

1. From your assessment recorded in the Analysis Table, is the child whose X ray appears in Figure 1.2 more or less physiologically mature than the standard for a 6-year-old? That is, is the skeletal age for the child of Figure 1.2 younger or older than 6.0 years? On what do you base your answer? Can you reach a conclusion about the chronological age of this child? Why or why not?

(Cont.)

2. From your assessment recorded in the Analysis Table, is the child whose X ray appears in Figure 1.3 more or less physiologically mature than the standard for a 6-year-old? What can you say about this child's chronological age in relation to skeletal age?

3. The standard X ray in Figure 1.1 depicts the skeletal development of a girl at 6.0 years of age. Would the X ray of an average boy at 6.0 years chronological age be likely to show more or less skeletal development? Why?

2

Assessing Growth Rate

Growth measures themselves do not reflect maturation, but often maturation can be implied by following the *rate* of growth. Growth rate can be illustrated by plotting the velocity curve for a curve depicting the *distance* or extent of growth. In this laboratory activity you will plot the velocity curve for a hypothetical distance curve for height. In this way, you can see how the velocity curve is obtained and how the two curves are related to one another.

Objective
- To understand the relationships between distance-of-growth curves and velocity curves.

Format   Independent work

Textbook Reading   "Plotting Growth" on pages 32 and 33

Procedure   1. Examine the distance curve in Figure 2.1. Calculate the increase in height between ages 6 and 7, then between ages 7 and 8, 8 and 9, and so on through age 21. For example, the increase in height between ages 8 and 9 is 1 cm.

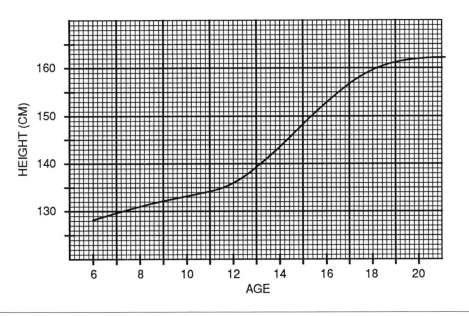

Figure 2.1

7

2. On the graph provided in Figure 2.2, plot points on a velocity curve at each age interval using the distance curve data calculated from Figure 2.1. Plot each age interval data point at the midpoint of the age range. For example, the one-centimeter increase in height between ages 6 and 7 is plotted at a point corresponding to 6.5 years on the velocity curve graph. The increase in height between ages 7 and 8 is plotted at age 7.5 years on the velocity graph, and so on. You will plot a total of fourteen points.

3. Connect the points on your velocity graph with a *smooth* curve.

Name _____ **Section** _____ **Date** _____

LABORATORY 2: ASSESSING GROWTH RATE
Velocity Curve Graph

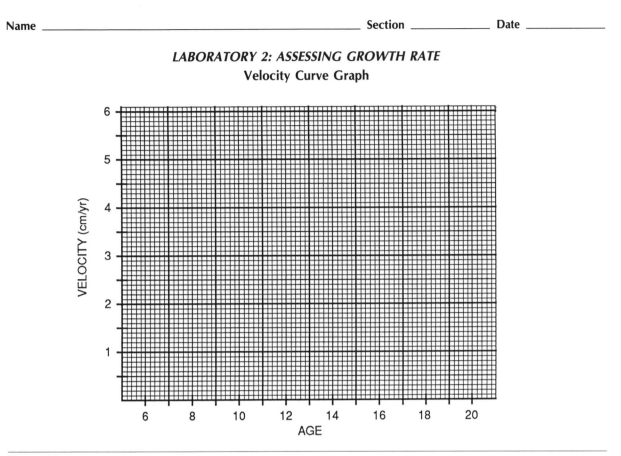

Figure 2.2

Discussion Questions

1. Describe what the distance curve tells you about the child's growth in height.

(Cont.)

2. Describe what the velocity curve you plotted tells about the child's rate of growth in height.

3. Are there peaks and valleys in your velocity curve? Where? What do these peaks and valleys tell you about the child's growth? What points on the distance curve correspond to the peaks and valleys in the velocity curve?

3

Measuring Extent of Growth

There are various measurements of growth, including height, weight, body part circumferences, and body lengths and breadths. Regularly recording such measurements is valuable for detecting deviations from normal growth, so that individuals can be referred as appropriate to health care professionals. Children also find it interesting to follow their own growth, to better understand the changes in their bodies and the general growth process. Implications about maturation can sometimes be made from growth measurements, which helps both teachers and children to set realistic expectations for skill performance.

Professionals who take growth measurements must be precise and accurate. Growth measurements must be taken consistently at specific sites using identical procedures, especially if they are to be compared to past or future recordings. Achieving this precision requires care and practice in measurement techniques. In this laboratory activity you will practice taking growth measurements, first on a classmate, then on a child. Some interesting measurements, such as the biacromial/biiliac breadth, also can be derived from direct growth measurements. This laboratory activity acquaints you with some of these calculated growth indicators as well as the basic growth measurements.

Objectives
- To learn to measure various body dimensions accurately and to practice taking these measurements.
- To derive other growth measurements from raw growth data.
- To compare an individual's growth to standard growth charts and tables.
- To relate growth measurements to maturation.

Format
With a partner in the laboratory, about 25 minutes. Then a visit to a clinical setting with your laboratory partner to measure a child, about 30 minutes.

Textbook Readings
"Growth Measures" on pages 21-30 and "Normal Postnatal Growth" on pages 44-56

Equipment Needed
- Stadiometer or long anthropometer to measure height (metric scale)
- Skinfold calipers
- Breadth or bow calipers (anthropometer; metric scale)
- Steel tape measure (metric scale)

Procedure

1. Practice taking growth measurements on a classmate (adult) as directed on the Growth Measures Data Sheet. It is useful to practice with the measuring instruments on cooperative subjects before working with children, who may be restless. If an anatomical skeleton is available, check the bony landmarks on the skeleton before attempting the breadth measurements on your classmate. You may also practice taking the measurements on the skeleton.

2. For consistency, take all ipsilateral measurements on the right side.

3. For circumference measurements, make sure the steel tape contacts the skin all the way around, but does not compress it. Place the zero mark at the subject's side so that you can easily read the final measurement while standing at the subject's side. Be sure the tape is right side up so that you will not have to read it upside down (a common source of error).

4. Take three measurements, then average them. Start from the beginning for each measurement; this increases the chances of accuracy. By doing so you will realize immediately if you have reversed a digit when recording the result or have let the instrument slip out of position, and so forth.

5. Record each measurement immediately: Don't trust your memory! Also, skinfold measurements may change if the caliper is left in place very long. If you work in groups of two or more, one person can take the measurement and call out the result. The other person can repeat the number aloud as it is written, and the one who took the measurement can check it on the instrument.

6. After measuring an adult, repeat each measurement on a child (between 3 and 10 years of age preferably). It is best to measure a child of the same sex as your laboratory partner. (Later you will compare certain measurements on the adult and the child, and these comparisons are best made between members of the same sex.)

7. After recording all of the growth measurements, obtain the results and figure the calculations listed in the Results and Calculations Table.

Growth Measures Data Sheet (Adult)

Subject _____ Sex **M** **F** **Birthdate** ___/___/___

Measurement	Trial 1	Trial 2	Trial 3	Average
Standing height (stature) Barefoot, weight on both feet, heels together, arms at side, head up				cm
Sitting height Height sitting on stool with thighs parallel to floor, hips against wall or instrument, head up. Subtract stool height unless instrument can be placed on stool.				cm
Weight Minimal clothing, shoes off, standing in center of platform				kg
Head circumference Above eyebrows, horizontal plane				cm
For the next two measurements, measure halfway between olecranon (elbow) and acromion process and mark[a] Upper arm circumference At mark, arm abducted, elbow flexed, forearm supinated, fist clenched, tape measure perpendicular to long axis of arm				cm
Triceps skinfold Back of arm at mark, relaxed arm at side; raise a vertical fold of skin just above mark, and apply caliper at mark midway between crest and base of fold				mm
Calf skinfold Place a mark on the inside of the calf (medial) at the level of maximum calf circumference; raise a vertical fold of skin just above the mark, and apply caliper at mark midway between crest and base of fold				mm
Biacromial (shoulder) breadth Weight evenly distributed on feet; palpate for acromion process; from back of subject place instrument on lateral edge of acromion process; have subject exhale and relax				cm
Biiliac (hip) breadth Palpate for iliac crest from back of subject, and place instrument on lateral edge of iliac crest; skin and adipose tissue may be compressed by applying pressure				cm

[a]Upper arm circumference is often taken at the largest part of the arm, but the midpoint measurement is needed here for a later calculation.

Growth Measures Data Sheet (Child)

Subject _____ Sex   M   F   Birthdate ____/____/____

Measurement	Trial 1	Trial 2	Trial 3	Average
Standing height (stature) Barefoot, weight on both feet, heels together, arms at side, head up (you may hold child at the jaw)				cm
Sitting height Height sitting on stool with thighs parallel to floor, hips against wall or instrument, head up. Subtract stool height unless instrument can be placed on stool.				cm
Weight Minimal clothing, shoes off, standing in center of platform				kg
Head circumference Above eyebrows, horizontal plane				cm
For the next two measurements, measure halfway between olecranon (elbow) and acromion process and mark[a] Upper arm circumference At mark, arm abducted, elbow flexed, forearm supinated, fist clenched, tape measure perpendicular to long axis of arm				cm
Triceps skinfold Back of arm at mark, relaxed arm at side; raise a vertical fold of skin just above mark, and apply caliper at mark midway between crest and base of fold				mm
Calf skinfold Place a mark on the inside of the calf (medial) at the level of maximum calf circumference; raise a vertical fold of skin just above the mark, and apply caliper at mark midway between crest and base of fold				mm
Biacromial (shoulder) breadth Weight evenly distributed on feet; palpate for acromion process; from back of subject place instrument on lateral edge of acromion process; have subject exhale and relax				cm
Biiliac (hip) breadth Palpate for iliac crest from back of subject, and place instrument on lateral edge of iliac crest; skin and adipose tissue may be compressed by applying pressure				cm

[a]Upper arm circumference is often taken at the largest part of the arm, but the midpoint measurement is needed here for a later calculation.

Name _____ **Section** _____ **Date** _____

LABORATORY 3: MEASURING EXTENT OF GROWTH
Results and Calculations Table

Result/Calculation	Adult	Child
From the birthdate, compute the *decimal age*. Divide number of months since last birthdate by 12.	years	years
Approximate the *height percentile* for age from Figure 2.2a and b in the textbook. Use age eighteen for adults.	%ile	%ile
Approximate the *weight percentile* for age from Figure 2.3a and b in the textbook. Use age eighteen for adults.	%ile	%ile
Approximate the *head circumference percentile* (for children only) using the table in Appendix A.	%ile	%ile
Calculate the *biacromial/biiliac breadth ratio*. $\dfrac{\text{Biacromial breadth}}{\text{Biiliac breadth}} \times 100 =$ _____ $\times\ 100 =$		
Calculate the *lean circumference of the upper arm*. $C - \pi\,(s) =$ _____ cm $-\ 3.14\,($ _____ cm$) =$ where $\pi = 3.14$, C is the upper arm circumference in centimeters, and s is the triceps skinfold in centimeters (remember to convert from millimeters)	cm	cm
Calculate the *functional leg length*. Functional leg length $=$ Standing height $-$ Sitting height	cm	cm
Calculate the *legs' percentage of height*. $\dfrac{\text{Leg length}}{\text{Standing height}} \times 100 =$ _____ $\times\ 100 =$	%	%
Calculate the *percentage of body fat*. Triceps skinfold (mm) $+$ Calf skinfold (mm) $=$	mm	mm
Percentage of body fat from Figure 3.1 (Note: This estimation is not accurate for adults.)	%	%

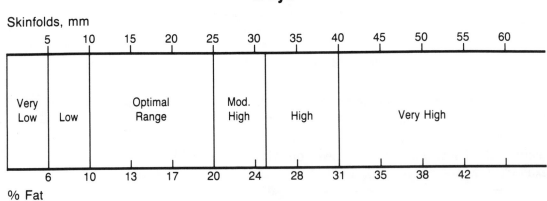

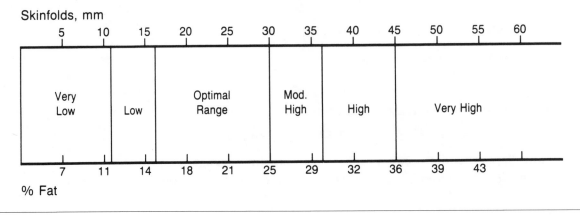

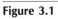

Figure 3.1

Name _____ Section _____ Date _____

Discussion Questions

1. Consider the percentile scores obtained on the child. What can you conclude about the child's maturation (as different than growth)? Why?

2. Compare the biacromial/biiliac breadth ratios of the adult and the child you measured. Do the same for the legs' percentage of total height. What can you conclude from this comparison about the growth of body proportions? Consider the age of the child and whether the adult and child you measured were of the same sex.

(Cont.)

3. Is more of the upper arm's circumference fat or lean tissue? Compare the lean circumference measures of the upper arm for the adult with those of the child. What can you conclude about the growth of lean and fat tissue from this comparison? Consider the sex of your subjects as well as the age of the child.

4. Consider the estimated percentage of body fat of the child. Is this child above, below, or at the average percentage of body fat? What feedback would you give this child regarding his or her percentage of body fat?

PART

II

Assessing Early Motor Development

A preferred method of assessing early motor development is to note the acquisition of new motor skills. In a few short years the infant/toddler acquires a whole repertoire of skills leading to upright locomotion and precise manipulation. Many of the basic motor skills—the *motor milestones*—are acquired in a precise, fixed order. The age at which they are acquired, though, is variable. Normal development is characterized by acquisition of skills within a known age range, and delayed development is suspected if acquisition of motor skills is late. Motor development can be assessed by comparing the age at which specific skills are acquired to norms for the age group.

Comparison of a child's age at skill onset to norms is only one use of information about the acquisition of new skills. Parents and educators can facilitate skill development after identifying skills already achieved and those the infant/toddler is on the verge of mastering. An assessment scale designed to provide this information is termed a *criterion-referenced* scale.

In laboratory activities 4 and 5 you will observe motor skills of an infant and a toddler. You will use a normative scale to assess the infant's skills and a criterion-referenced scale to gauge the toddler's skills. That is, you will determine whether the infant's skills are appropriate for his or her age, according to age norms; for the toddler, you will identify skills performed with competency, skills just emerging, and skills not yet exhibited. By completing the laboratory assignments you will gain experience with both types of scales while learning about the motor skills of infants and toddlers.

Observing the Motor Milestones

The rudimentary motor skills leading to locomotion and visually guided reaching are acquired in a consistent sequence, making it possible to identify a common age range for acquisition of each skill. Of course, there is some variation in the rate of appearance of the motor milestones. The rate of physical maturation and a variety of environmental factors play roles in individual variability. Several normative scales exist for comparing an infant to the average age and range of ages when a given skill is acquired by normally developing infants. Infants who acquire skills late thus can be identified and monitored by professionals.

In this activity you will observe the motor development of an infant under 1 year of age and compare him or her to a normative scale adapted from the Bayley Scale and to a scale for grasping development. Remember that every great athlete started by acquiring these same rudimentary skills.

Objectives
- To observe the motor milestone skills in an infant under 1 year of age.
- To assess the rate of motor development in an infant by comparison to a normative scale.

Format   Clinical setting, about 30 minutes

Textbook Reading   "Motor Milestones" on pages 83-90

Equipment Needed
- A toy ring
- A building block

Procedure
1. Your instructor will arrange for you to work with an infant.
2. Obtain the background and general information, particularly age. Enter "NA" (not available) for any information you cannot get.
3. Use the Observation Scale for Infant Development first. Starting with the first item, position the infant as directed. Check "Pass" if the infant exhibits the behavior and "Fail" if not. Enter an "R" for refused or "RBC" for reported by caretaker under "Other" if appropriate. You need not administer the entire scale. If an infant fails several items in a row and is obviously developmentally younger than the age range for an item, you may stop.

4. Proceed to the Observation Scale for Grasping Development. Position the infant upright in front of a table or tray. Place a building block on the table. Observe how the infant grasps the block; repeat this several times. The drawings on page 89, Figure 3.3, of the textbook might be helpful.

Name _____ Section _____ Date _____

LABORATORY 4: OBSERVING THE MOTOR MILESTONES
Data Sheet

Background and General Information

Today's date _____ Infant's birthdate _____ Infant's age _____._____ months

APGAR score at birth _____ Weight at birth _____

Was infant full-term or premature? Full-term _____ Premature _____ No. of weeks _____

Special medical problems _____

_____

Is parent/caretaker present?   Y   N   Time of day _____

How does infant react to you (cries, smiles, etc.)? _____

Hours since last feeding _____ Next feeding expected at _____

Hours since last nap _____ Next nap expected at _____

Clothing that may restrict the infant's movement _____

_____

Infant's general level of alertness/activity _____

Observation Scale for Infant Development

	Pass	Fail	Other	Behavior	Average age (months)	Age range (months)
1.	____	____	____	When held upright, lifts head	0.1	
2.	____	____	____	When prone, makes crawling moves	0.4	.1– 3.0
3.	____	____	____	When supine, holds toy ring	0.8	.3– 3.0
4.	____	____	____	When supine, thrusts arms in play	0.8	.3– 2.0
5.	____	____	____	When supine, thrusts legs in play	0.8	.3– 2.0
6.	____	____	____	Held upright, keeps head erect	1.6	.7– 4.0
7.	____	____	____	Supine, turns from side to back	1.8	.7– 5.0
8.	____	____	____	Prone, elevates self by arms	2.1	.7– 5.0
9.	____	____	____	Sits with support on hard surface	2.3	1.0– 5.0
10.	____	____	____	Upright, holds head steady	2.5	1.0– 5.0
11.	____	____	____	Hands predominantly open	2.7	.7– 6.0
12.	____	____	____	Sits with slight support on hard surface	3.8	2.0– 6.0
13.	____	____	____	Supine, turns from back to side	4.4	2.0– 7.0
14.	____	____	____	Makes effort to sit with help	4.8	3.0– 8.0
15.	____	____	____	Pulls to sitting with help	5.3	4.0– 8.0
16.	____	____	____	Sits alone momentarily on hard surface	5.3	4.0– 8.0
17.	____	____	____	Reaches with one arm	5.4	4.0– 8.0
18.	____	____	____	Rotates wrist	5.7	4.0– 8.0
19.	____	____	____	Sits alone thirty seconds or more	6.0	5.0– 8.0
20.	____	____	____	When supine, rolls from back to front	6.4	4.0–10.0
21.	____	____	____	Sits alone steadily, hard surface	6.6	5.0– 9.0

(Cont.)

LABORATORY 4 (Cont.)

Observation Scale for Infant Development

	Pass	Fail	Other	Behavior	Average age (months)	Age range (months)
22.				Locomotor progression:	7.1	5.0–11.0
	___	___	___	Moves on abdomen		
	___	___	___	Moves on hands and knees		
	___	___	___	Moves on hands and feet		
	___	___	___	Sits and hitches		
23.	___	___	___	When upright, early stepping movements	7.4	5.0–11.0
24.	___	___	___	Pulls to standing position	8.1	5.0–12.0
25.	___	___	___	Raises to sitting position	8.3	6.0–11.0
26.	___	___	___	Stands up by furniture	8.6	6.0–12.0
27.	___	___	___	Stepping movements	8.8	6.0–12.0
28.	___	___	___	Walks with help	9.6	7.0–12.0
29.	___	___	___	Sits down from standing	9.6	7.0–14.0
30.	___	___	___	Stands alone	11.0	9.0–16.0
31.	___	___	___	Walks alone	11.7	9.0–17.0
32.	___	___	___	Stands up from floor	12.6	9.0–18.0
33.	___	___	___	Throws ball	13.3	9.0–18.0

Note. Adapted from the Motor Scale of the "Bayley Scales of Infant Development." Copyright 1969 by the Psychological Corporation, 555 Academic Court, San Antonio, TX 78204-0952. Reprinted by permission. If you assess an infant in an official capacity, you should obtain the official Bayley Scale from the Psychological Corporation.

Name _____ Section _____ Date _____

Observation Scale for Grasping Development

Directions: Place a block on the table in front of the upright infant.

	Pass	Fail	Type of grasp	Average age (months)	Age range (months)
1.	____	____	Makes no contact with block	4.0	4.0– 8.0
2.	____	____	Makes contact with block but does not secure it	5.0	4.0–13.0
3.	____	____	Primitive squeeze: Thrusts hand beyond block, then pulls it toward self until squeezed against body or other hand	5.0	5.0– 6.0
4.	____	____	Squeeze grasp: Hand approaches from side, fingers close on block to press it against heel of palm; cannot raise block	6.0	5.0– 8.0
5.	____	____	Hand grasp: Hand is brought down on block, and block is squeezed against heel of palm with fingers on far side, thumb on adjacent side	7.0	5.0–13.0
6.	____	____	Palm grasp: Hand is brought down on block as above, but thumb is placed on near surface to oppose the fingers	7.0	5.0–10.0
7.	____	____	Superior palm: Thumb side of the hand is brought down on the block with the thumb on the near side and the first two fingers on the far side	8.0	7.0–13.0
8.	____	____	Inferior forefinger: As above but block is not held against palm; grasp maintained with fingers	9.0	8.0–13.0
9.	____	____	Forefinger: Block is grasped with fingertips, thumb opposing first two or three fingers	13.0	9.0–13.0
10.	____	____	Superior forefinger: As forefinger grasp, but hand does not contact table; block is lifted deftly after grasp	13.0	13.0+

Note.   From *Genetic Psychology Monographs*, **10**, p. 107, 1931. Reprinted with permission of the Helen Dwight Reid Educational Foundation. Published by Heldref Publications, 4000 Albemarle St., N.W., Washington, D.C. 20016. Copyright © 1931.

Discussion Questions

1. How far has the infant progressed along the sequence of motor milestones? Does the baby's chronological age match the average age and age range for the skills you observed? What can you conclude about the infant's motor development?

(Cont.)

2. When the baby was lifted from a back-lying position, what was the response of the head? Could the baby sit independently or with support? What postural responses did the infant make in the sitting position? Could the baby stand with support or alone? What postural responses did the infant make when standing?

3. Did you observe one or several types of grasp? If several, which was used most often?

4. Does the infant's chronological age match the average age and age range of her or his predominant grasp? What can you conclude about the baby's grasping development?

5. How did circumstances such as the infant's reaction to you or the time lapse since the last feeding or nap affect performance of the infant's motor skills? Did the baby's clothing seem to restrict the execution of any skills?

6. Given that this might have been your first observation of infant motor development and that you observed the infant only briefly, how confident are you that your results are accurate? What would you say in explaining your results to the infant's caretaker?

5

Observing Toddler Motor Development

A normative scale such as that used in Laboratory 4 is useful in showing how a baby performs in comparison to a reference group of infants. An alternative purpose in assessing skill acquisition during early childhood is to determine whether a child can do a certain skill. When this is the goal it is appropriate to use a criterion-referenced assessment scale. The child's performance is compared to a predetermined level of mastery, rather than to the scores of other children. This assessment permits parents and educators to design an instructional program aimed at fostering the further mastery of basic skills.

Two sections of the Geismar-Ryan Infant-Toddler Developmental Checklist are used here to give you experience with a criterion-referenced scale. One section assesses gross-motor and the other fine-motor activities. You will identify those skills a child performs with competence, those skills in which no competency is demonstrated, and those skills in which competency is just emerging. Skills in the latter two categories would be the basis for planning learning activities for the child, were this your purpose.

Objectives
- To observe motor development in early childhood.
- To use a criterion-referenced scale for assessment of motor development.

Format Clinical setting, about 1 hour

Textbook Readings "Skill Refinement" on pages 74 and 75 and "Critical Periods" on pages 90-93

Equipment Needed
- Small toy
- Small chair
- Small rocking chair
- Push cart
- Push/pull toy
- Balance beam

- Ball
- Cheerios cereal
- Small bottle
- Crayon and paper
- String and beads
- Pegboard and pegs

- Building blocks
- Puzzle or formboard
- Cardboard book
- Safety scissors
- Bowl and jars with lids

Procedure
1. Your instructor will make arrangements for you to visit a preschool program or nursery school. You should administer this scale to a toddler over 1 year of age but younger than 5. Ask your instructor whether the equipment needed is available at the school or if you must bring some items.
2. Obtain as much general and background information on the child as possible.

3. Review the scale beforehand. Become familiar with the tasks so that you can instruct the child, set up equipment, or provide opportunity for the child to demonstrate the behavior.

4. Items at the beginning of each scale are easier and therefore more appropriate for younger children, while later items are more difficult and more suitable for older children. You may skip items obviously easy for the child. For example, items 1 to 4 on the gross-motor section might be skipped if you are working with a 4-year-old.

5. Each item is preceded by a 1—2—3 scale. After setting up the opportunity for a child to perform an item, circle the number most accurately representing the child's level of ability:

   1 = Competency not demonstrated.
   2 = Competency is emerging (demonstrated inconsistently and/or much assistance needed).
   3 = Competency demonstrated regularly.

6. Comments are frequently used with this assessment to reflect an individual's uniqueness. If you would like to comment on performance of an item, mark it with a "C" and number it accordingly on a blank sheet.

Name _____ Section _____ Date _____

LABORATORY 5: OBSERVING TODDLER MOTOR DEVELOPMENT
Data Sheet

Child's first name _____ Sex _____

Birthdate _____ Observation date _____ Decimal age _____ . _____ years

Time of day _____ Time until next meal _____ Time until next nap _____

Special medical problems _____

The Geismar-Ryan Infant-Toddler Developmental Checklist

Gross-Motor Development

1—2—3   1 Reaches for toy or person when lying on stomach

1—2—3   2 Sits unsupported momentarily (30 seconds)

1—2—3   3 Assumes quadruped position and rocks on all fours

1—2—3   4 Assumes quadruped position and crawls

1—2—3   5 Demonstrates large muscle skills in the prewalking area, as in
    Sitting alone
    Pulling to stand
    Lowering self to floor
    Cruising by holding on to furniture
    Taking steps when supported

1—2—3   6 Stands alone

1—2—3   7 Uses mobility skills to actively explore environment, as in
    Walking alone
    Crawling up steps
    Getting around barriers

1—2—3   8 Walks well (stops, starts, turns)

1—2—3   9 Demonstrates some variety of walking skills, as in
    Walking sideways and backwards
    Walking up and down stairs holding on
    Some beginning "running"

1—2—3 10 Squats in play and resumes standing position

1—2—3 11 Seats self in small chair

1—2—3 12 Demonstrates some coordinated use of large-motor skills with a variety of equipment, as in
    Walking with a push/pull toy
    Pushing a cart
    Rocking on a chair
    Going down a slide

1—2—3 13 Demonstrates some balance in walking, jumping, and hopping, as in
    Balancing on one foot with help
    Jumping in place with two feet
    Walking on a balance beam with help

1—2—3 14 Kicks ball forward

1—2—3 15 Throws ball forward 5 to 7 feet

1—2—3 16 Uses simple motor skills socially, as in simple games of "Ring-Around-a-Rosy" or "London Bridge"

(Cont.)

LABORATORY 5 (Cont.)

Gross-Motor Development

1—2—3   17 Coordinates series of physical skills in play, as in
                Lifting, carrying, and arranging large hollow blocks
                Carrying objects while climbing

Fine-Motor Development

Thumb/finger opposition (pincer grasp)

1—2—3   1 Rakes or scoops up Cheerio and attains it
1—2—3   2 Has complete thumb opposition on cube
1—2—3   3 Uses inferior pincer grasp with Cheerio
1—2—3   4 Uses neat pincer grasp with Cheerio
1—2—3   5 Releases Cheerio into small bottle

Crayon use/scribbling

1—2—3   6 Attempts to scribble by holding crayon to paper
1—2—3   7 Holds crayon adaptively
1—2—3   8 Scribbles spontaneously
1—2—3   9 Imitates crayon strokes (vertical and circular scribble)
1—2—3   10 Holds crayon with fingers
1—2—3   11 Scribbles with circular motion
1—2—3   12 Copies a circle already drawn

Pegboard use

1—2—3   13 Pulls pegs out of pegboard
1—2—3   14 Pokes with isolated finger
1—2—3   15 Places one or two pegs in pegboard with help
1—2—3   16 Places two to six pegs in pegboard without help

Building

1—2—3   17 Transfers toy from hand to hand
1—2—3   18 Drops a block with voluntary release
1—2—3   19 Builds two-cube tower
1—2—3   20 Builds tower of two to six cubes
1—2—3   21 Builds tower and other constructions of more than six cubes

Formboard/puzzles

1—2—3   22 Places round form(s) in formboard
1—2—3   23 Completes three-piece formboard or puzzle

Other

1—2—3   24 Turns pages of cardboard book
1—2—3   25 Removes cover from small box and unscrews jar lids
1—2—3   26 Attempts to fold paper imitatively
1—2—3   27 Cuts with scissors
1—2—3   28 Strings beads

Note. The complete Geismar-Ryan Infant-Toddler Developmental Checklist can be obtained from Dr. Lori Geismar-Ryan, Childhood Education Department, University of Missouri-St. Louis, 8001 Natural Bridge Road, St. Louis, MO 63121.

Name _____ **Section** _____ **Date** _____

Discussion Questions

1. For each aspect of development listed, summarize skills that the toddler can demonstrate competently.

   Gross-motor

   Fine-motor

2. For each aspect of development listed, identify emerging skills:

   Gross-motor

   Fine-motor

3. What types of activities would be helpful for this toddler to gain competence in the emerging skills you identified?

   Gross-motor

   Fine-motor

(Cont.)

Discussion Questions on Laboratories 4 and 5

1. How is a normative scale (Laboratory 4) different from a criterion-referenced scale (Laboratory 5)?

2. What are the advantages and disadvantages of each type of scale?

3. Which scale did you prefer using? Why?

PART

III

Assessment of the Basic Motor Skills

The sequence of skill acquisition was described for several of the basic skills in chapter 4 of the textbook. Developmental change for most skills was discussed in terms of developmental steps or levels for each of the body components involved. Categorizing performers using those steps is a means of assessing their skill development. For example, physical education teachers who want to evaluate the basic motor development of students can do so by identifying the developmental level at which they are performing. This, of course, is a qualitative rather than a quantitative assessment of skill.

The ability to assess qualitative development must be practiced repeatedly with an established and systematic observation plan. The next series of laboratory activities is designed to provide you with, first, an observation plan, and second, an opportunity to practice assessing development of several basic skills. Sequential, still pictures are provided to let you practice, with plenty of time to find the important criteria and make your decision. Still photographs often lack some action that you need to make a categorization, but this will be valuable initial practice. Your instructor may then provide you with a videotape or film, which is more realistic practice, but still more difficult than still photographs. Finally, you

should practice assessing performers in a realistic setting. You will likely find this challenging because the movements you will be looking for occur so quickly.

The more practice observation and assessment you do, the better you will become. Your instructor will tell you whether to observe all or just some of the skills in Laboratories 6 through 11. At the least you should observe one continuous locomotor skill (running or hopping) and one ballistic skill (throwing or striking). Whichever skills you are assigned, read the first laboratory exercise on running, because it gives more detailed instructions than the others.

It may save time to do all of your independent work in Laboratories 6 through 11 first, then to watch all videotapes or films your instructor provides in one or two sittings. Likewise you probably will want to make your "live" observation of all of the skills assigned to you in one session. It is interesting to observe an individual on several skills to determine whether she or he is at approximately equal developmental levels.

You may find the observation plans and checklists useful in a variety of settings even after completing this course. You might want to laminate the observation plans and extra checklists provided in Appendix B.

LABORATORY

6

Assessing the Developmental Level of Running

In the first of this series of laboratory activities you will observe and assess running. Be sure you are familiar with the developmental changes in running described on pages 104-107 of your textbook. Recall that developmental steps for running have not been validated, hence the observation plan for running that follows in this laboratory is not as precise as those for some other skills.

Objectives
- To become familiar with an observation plan for running.
- To practice assessment of running development with photographs, videotapes, or films.
- To plan an observation of running and to practice the assessment of runners in person.

Format
Independent work, about 20 minutes; class or free time to watch videotape or film, about 20 minutes; clinical setting to observe a runner in person, about 15 minutes.

Textbook Readings
"Running" on pages 104-107, "Observing Motor Skill Patterns" on pages 138 and 139, and "Quantitative Versus Qualitative Assessment" on pages 146-149

Procedure
1. Using the sequential still photos (Figures 6.1 and 6.2), follow the observation plan to assess each performer. As you categorize the leg and arm action of each, check the appropriate step on the checklist. Finally, enter the step number on the summary profile. You may want to place the checklist on a clipboard. If the photos do not provide enough information to decide between two levels, check and record both (e.g., 3/4) on the summary profile.

2. Your instructor may schedule you to watch a videotape or film of running performance. If you can show it in slow motion, that will be helpful for the first few performers. Thereafter, try to make your decisions at full-speed viewing. For at least one decision in the observation plan, you will have to wait for a rear angle on the videotape or film. Follow the observation plan and fill out the checklist as you did for the photos.

3. After your videotape assessment, your instructor might schedule (or have you schedule) a time to observe running in person. Try to observe at least two runners, including one who is not highly skilled. You may find it interesting to observe an older adult. Decide what instructions you will need to give the runners beforehand, and remember to move in order to observe from different angles. For running you will observe the limb or joint as directed by the observation plan for

several running strides. Once you can make a decision, observe the next limb or joint specified.

4. Your instructor may ask you for the results of your assessment of runners in the photographs and the videotape or film. Be ready to defend your decisions.

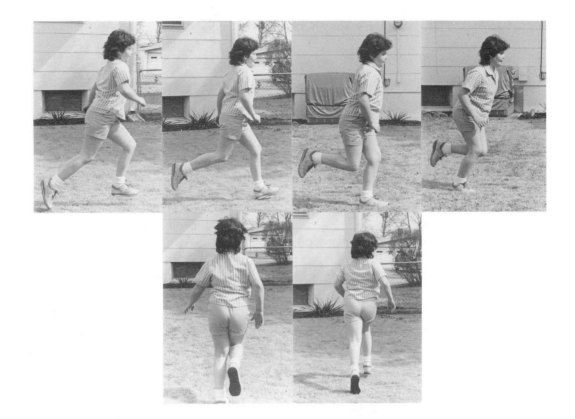

Figure 6.1.   CH, age 8.9 years, running.

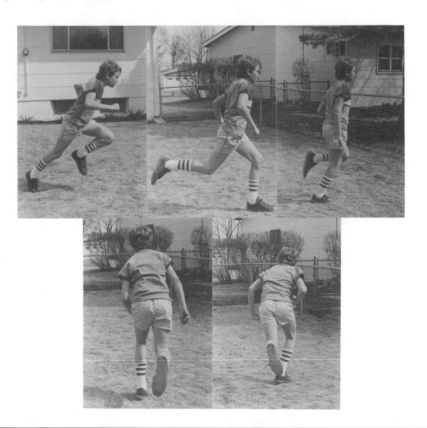

Figure 6.2.   MH, age 12.0 years, running.

OBSERVATION PLAN FOR RUNNING

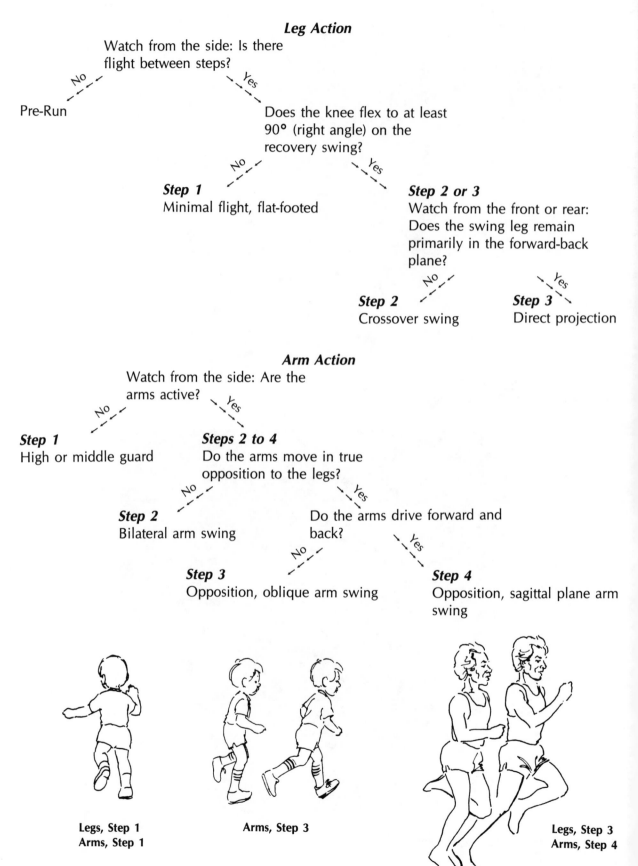

Leg Action

Watch from the side: Is there flight between steps?

No → **Pre-Run**

Yes → Does the knee flex to at least 90° (right angle) on the recovery swing?

No → **Step 1** Minimal flight, flat-footed

Yes → **Step 2 or 3** Watch from the front or rear: Does the swing leg remain primarily in the forward-back plane?

No → **Step 2** Crossover swing

Yes → **Step 3** Direct projection

Arm Action

Watch from the side: Are the arms active?

No → **Step 1** High or middle guard

Yes → **Steps 2 to 4** Do the arms move in true opposition to the legs?

No → **Step 2** Bilateral arm swing

Yes → Do the arms drive forward and back?

No → **Step 3** Opposition, oblique arm swing

Yes → **Step 4** Opposition, sagittal plane arm swing

Legs, Step 1
Arms, Step 1

Arms, Step 3

Legs, Step 3
Arms, Step 4

Name _____ Section _____ Date _____

LABORATORY 6: ASSESSING THE DEVELOPMENTAL LEVEL OF RUNNING

OBSERVATION CHECKLIST: *Running*

Observation number	1	2	3	4	5	6	7
Runner's name							
Runner's age							
Date							
Observation type[a]							
Component							
Leg action							
Pre-run							
Step 1. Minimal flight							
Step 2. Crossover swing							
Step 3. Direct projection							
Arm action							
Step 1. Middle guard							
Step 2. Bilateral arm swing							
Step 3. Oblique arm swing							
Step 4. Opposition, sagittal							
Summary profile							
Leg							
Arm							

[a]Codes for observation type: D = direct; P = photographs; F = film; V = video; s = slow motion.

Discussion Questions

1. Did you find instances where a performer was at a different level on a subsequent attempt of a skill? If so, describe them.

(Cont.)

2. Did an older child or adult perform at a lower level than someone younger? Describe any such instance.

3. Were any individuals at different levels for different body components? If so, describe.

4. How did your instructions make a difference in skill performance? How might different cue words elicit a more advanced performance level? In what body component(s)?

5. How might the task (for example, running versus sprinting) or the surroundings (for example, concrete surface versus grass) influence the level of performance? What might you change to elicit a more advanced level? State the body component and level involved.

6. What were the differences among the methods of observation (photos, slow-motion video, etc.)? Which method was the easiest and which the hardest? What are the disadvantages of each observation method in making an accurate assessment?

7

Assessing the Developmental Level of the Standing Long Jump

In this laboratory exercise you will observe and assess the standing long jump. The process is somewhat different than observing running. Running is repetitive; you can focus on a joint or limb, watch it for several strides, then make a decision. In contrast, a jumper executes only one standing long jump at a time. You will need to make a decision based on as few jumps as possible, before the jumper tires. Be sure to know both the developmental steps in Table 4.4 on pages 110 and 111 of your textbook and the observation plan. Then you will not "waste" jumps when you evaluate a jumper in person. You might be able to watch a body component (such as the legs) all the way through the jump. That is, you can watch that component during take-off, flight, and landing. This also will help you to complete your assessment quickly.

Objectives
- To learn an observation plan for the standing long jump.
- To practice categorizing jumpers into developmental levels, first with pictures, then videotape or film, and finally in person.
- To gain enough proficiency to categorize jumpers with minimal repetitions.

Format   Independent work, about 20 minutes; class or free time to watch videotapes or films, about 20 minutes; clinical setting to observe jumpers in person, about 15 minutes.

Textbook Reading   "Jumping" on pages 107-116

Procedure
1. Use the sequential photographs provided to categorize jumpers as you follow the observation plan. As you make a decision, check the appropriate box on the checklist; when you are finished, complete the summary profile.
2. If your instructor schedules you to watch a videotape or film, watch one or two jumpers in slow motion if possible. Following the observation guide, fill out the checklist as you did for the photographs. Finally, categorize one or two jumpers at full-speed viewing.
3. After practicing with photographs and videotape or film, observe jumpers in person. Decide what instructions to give beforehand, such as "start here" or "jump as far as you can." After an initial observation you might want to vary the instructions or the task to see if the jumper changes in any way. For example, you might ask a child to jump over a space you describe as a river or canyon.
4. Your instructor might ask you for the results of your assessment, or your class might discuss your results. Be ready to defend your decisions.

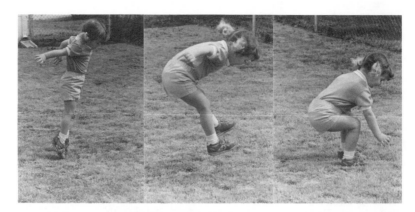

Figure 7.1. LH, age 3.2 years, long jumping.

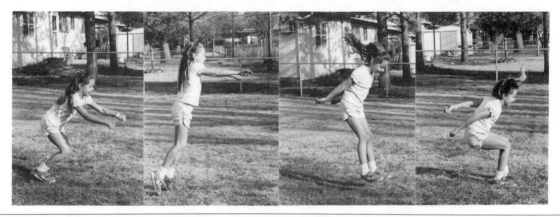

Figure 7.2. JS, age 7.9 years, long jumping.

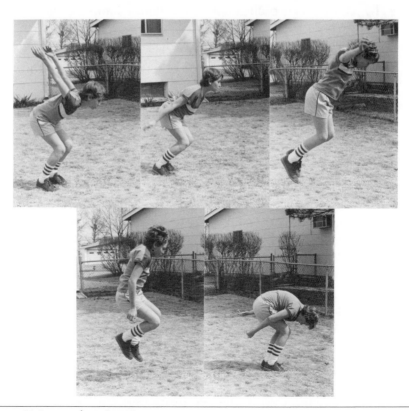

Figure 7.3. MH, age 12.0 years, long jumping.

OBSERVATION PLAN FOR THE STANDING LONG JUMP

Takeoff: Leg Action
Watch from the side: Do the
feet leave the ground together?

No   *Yes*

Step 1
Asymmetrical takeoff

Step 2 or 3
Are the hips and knees fully
extended at takeoff?

No   *Yes*

Step 2
Symmetrical, partial extension

Step 3
Symmetrical, extension

Takeoff: Trunk Action
Is the trunk more or less than
30° from vertical at takeoff?

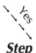

30°

Less   *More*

Step 1 or 2
Is the neck flexed or aligned?

No   *Yes*

Step 3 or 4
Is the neck aligned with the
trunk or extended?

No   *Yes*

Step 1
Less than 30°,
head back

Step 2
Less than 30°,
head flexed or
aligned

Step 3
More than 30°,
neck flexed

Step 4
More than 30°,
head aligned or
extended

Takeoff: Arm Action
Are the arms active; if so, do
they move symmetrically?

No ↙   ↘ Yes

Step 1
Arms inactive or asymmetrical

Steps 2 to 5
Do the arms move down and
back or do they move to the
side or front?

Down and Back ↙   ↘ Sideward or Forward

Step 2
Arms wing

Steps 3 to 5
Do the arms move out to the
side (abduct) or move forward?

Abduct ↙   ↘ Forward

Step 3
Arms abduct (high or middle
guard)

Do the arms move forward to
about shoulder level or overhead
(forming straight line with trunk)?

Shoulder level ↙   ↘ Overhead

Step 4
Arms forward, partial stretch

Step 5
Arms forward, full stretch

Arms abducted

Trunk lean less than 30°

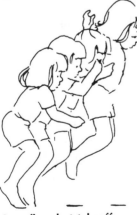

Legs flexed at takeoff

Toes pulled off ground

Step 1, Legs
Step 2, Trunk
Step 3, Arms

Trunk inclined more than 30°

Neck aligned

Arms in winging posture

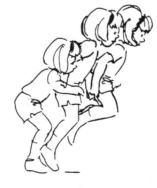

Knees and hips still flexed at takeoff

Step 2, Legs
Step 4, Trunk
Step 2, Arms

Neck is aligned

Deep preparatory crouch

Arms come forward

Hips and knees fully extended

Feet leave ground together

Step 3, Legs
Step 4, Trunk
Step 5, Arms

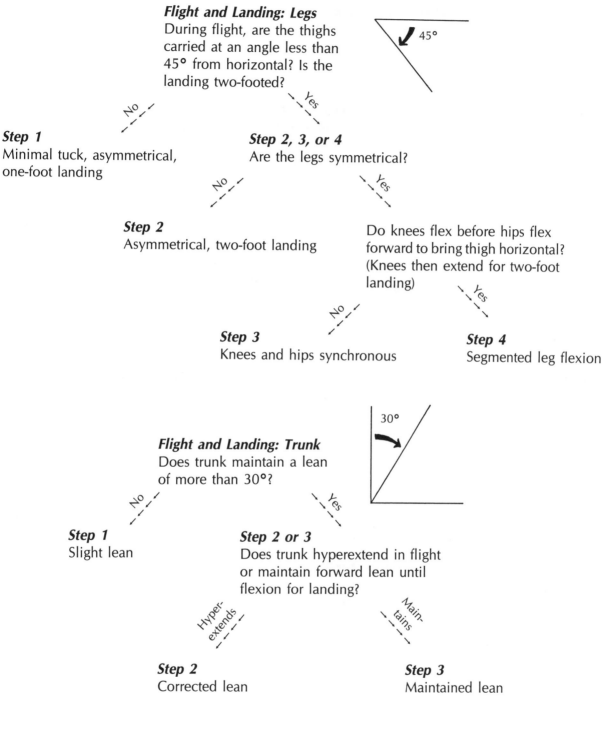

Flight and Landing: Legs
During flight, are the thighs carried at an angle less than 45° from horizontal? Is the landing two-footed?

45°

No

Yes

Step 1
Minimal tuck, asymmetrical, one-foot landing

Step 2, 3, or 4
Are the legs symmetrical?

No

Yes

Step 2
Asymmetrical, two-foot landing

Do knees flex before hips flex forward to bring thigh horizontal? (Knees then extend for two-foot landing)

Yes

No

Step 3
Knees and hips synchronous

Step 4
Segmented leg flexion

Flight and Landing: Trunk
Does trunk maintain a lean of more than 30°?

30°

No

Yes

Step 1
Slight lean

Step 2 or 3
Does trunk hyperextend in flight or maintain forward lean until flexion for landing?

Hyper-extends

Main-tains

Step 2
Corrected lean

Step 3
Maintained lean

Flight and Landing: Arms
Are the arms symmetrical?

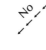
No

Yes

Step 1
Asymmetrical

Steps 2 to 4
Do arms wing (move backward)
in flight and parachute (move
forward) for landing or do they
remain forward/sideward?

Wing

Forward/
Sideward

Step 2
Winging

Step 3 or 4
Are the arms overhead, then
reaching forward for landing?

No

Yes

Step 3
High or middle guard

Step 4
Arms overhead, reach forward
for landing

Arms extended overhead at takeoff

Trunk flexes

Arms reach forward at landing

Arms still winging, trunk hyperextends

Arms laterally rotate

Arms parachute

Arms parachute

Trunk flexes

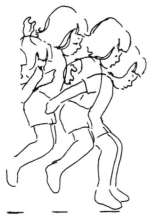

Knee flexion leads hip flexion

Knees and hips flex together in flight

Knees extend   Two-foot landing

Step 1, Legs
Step 1, Trunk
Step 3, Arms

Step 3, Legs
Step 2, Trunk
Step 2, Arms

Step 4, Legs
Step 3, Trunk
Step 4, Arms

Name _____ **Section** _____ **Date** _____

LABORATORY 7: ASSESSING THE DEVELOPMENTAL LEVEL OF THE STANDING LONG JUMP

OBSERVATION CHECKLIST: *Jumping*

Observation number	1	2	3	4	5	6	7
Jumper's name							
Jumper's age							
Date							
Observation type[a]							
Component							
Takeoff							
Leg							
Step 1. Asymmetrical							
Step 2. Symmetrical, bent							
Step 3. Symmetrical, full extension							
Trunk							
Step 1. Less than 30°, Neck hyperextended							
Step 2. Neck flexed/aligned							
Step 3. 30°, Neck flexed							
Step 4. 30°, Neck aligned							
Arm							
Step 1. Opposition							
Step 2. Winging							
Step 3. Guard							
Step 4. Arms flex							
Step 5. Arms flex, overhead							

[a]Codes for observation type: D = direct; P = photographs; F = film; V = video; s = slow motion.

(Cont.)

LABORATORY 7 (Cont.)

Observation number	1	2	3	4	5	6	7
Component							
Flight/landing							
Leg							
Step 1. One-foot landing							
Step 2. Asymmetrical, two-foot landing							
Step 3. Hip, knees flex together							
Step 4. Knees, then hips, flex							
Trunk							
Step 1. Less than 30°							
Step 2. 30°, Hyperextended							
Step 3. 30°, Flexes							
Arm							
Step 1. Opposition							
Step 2. Winging							
Step 3. Guard/windmill							
Step 4. Reach forward							
Summary profile							
Takeoff							
Leg							
Trunk							
Arm							
Flight/landing							
Leg							
Trunk							
Arm							

ᵃCodes for observation type: D = direct; P = photographs; F = film; V = video; s = slow motion.

Name _____ Section _____ Date _____

Discussion Questions

1. Did you find instances where a performer was at different levels during a series of jumps? If so, describe them.

2. Did an older child or adult perform at a lower level than someone younger? Describe any such instance.

3. Were any individuals at different levels for different body components? If so, describe.

(Cont.)

4. How did your instructions make a difference in skill performance? How might different cue words elicit a more advanced performance level? In what body component(s)?

5. How might the task (for example, jumping versus jumping as far as possible) or the surroundings (for example, concrete surface versus grass) influence the level of performance? What might you change to elicit a more advanced level? State the body component and level involved.

6. If you completed Laboratory 6, did it take you longer to assess a repetitive skill such as running or a discrete skill such as jumping?

8

Assessing the Developmental Level of Hopping

This laboratory experience on the development of hopping will proceed like the previous laboratories. Categorizing hoppers into developmental levels is easier than running, even though both are continuous locomotor skills, because the developmental steps for hopping have been partially validated. It is important to study Table 4.5 on pages 116 and 117 of the textbook before attempting this laboratory activity. There is not enough time during your observation to review—the observation plan assumes your knowledge of hopping.

Objectives
- To become familiar with an observation plan for hopping.
- To practice assessment of hopping using illustrations and videotapes or films.
- To learn how to position oneself to observe the critical features of hopping.

Format
Independent work, about 20 minutes; class or free time to watch videotape or film, about 20 minutes; clinical setting to observe hoppers in person, about 15 minutes.

Textbook Reading
"Hopping" on pages 116-120

Procedure
1. As with previous laboratories on the basic skills, conduct your initial assessments using the accompanying pictures.
2. Always use the observation plan as a guide. When you reach a decision on the leg action, then arm action, of the hopper, mark the appropriate box on the checklist. Finally, enter the step number on the summary profile.
3. Continue your observation practice by viewing a videotape or film of hoppers. If possible, categorize one or two hoppers from slow-motion viewing, then one or two at full speed.
4. Categorize one or two children in person. You might also observe adults to determine whether they have reached the highest developmental steps. Remember to plan your instructions ahead of time and to move around during observation to view from the best angle.
5. Be prepared to defend your decisions in a class discussion.

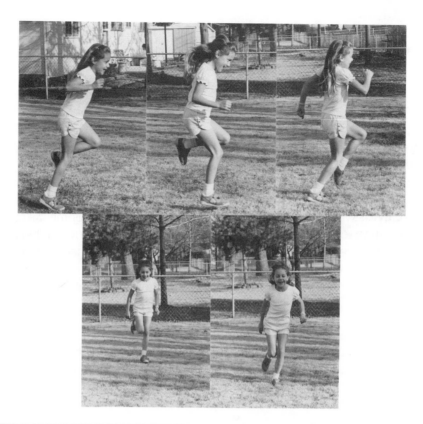

Figure 8.1. JS, age 7.9 years, hopping.

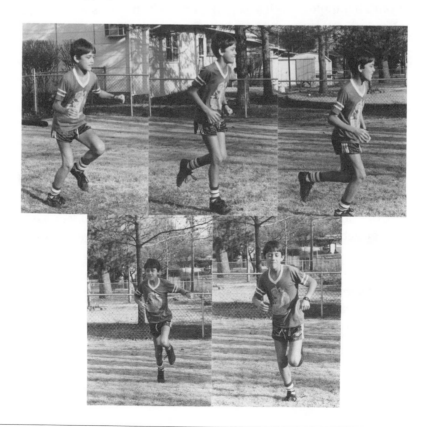

Figure 8.2. KS, age 10.2 years, hopping.

OBSERVATION PLAN FOR HOPPING

Leg Action
Focus on the swing leg from
the side: Is it active?

No / *Yes*

Step 1 or 2
Focus on the support leg: Does
it extend at takeoff to project
the body upward?

Step 3 or 4
Does the swing leg swing behind
the support leg? Look at the
support leg: Does the weight
shift to the ball of the support
foot before extension at takeoff?

No / *Yes*

No / *Yes*

Step 1
Momentary flight

Step 2
Fall and catch

Step 3
Projected takeoff

Step 4
Projection delay,
swing leg leads

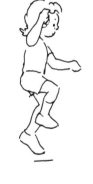

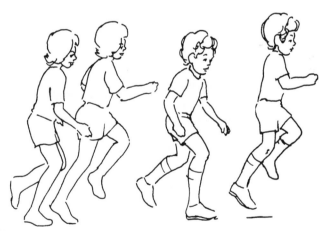

Minimal extension at takeoff

High, inactive swing leg

Step 2

Takeoff leg is extending

Swing leg leads

Support leg pulled up from floor

Step 3

Swing leg is seen fully behind support leg

Step 1

Support leg will fully extend at takeoff

Step 4

Arm Action
Move to watch the arms from
the side and the front: Is arm
action bilateral or opposing?

Bilateral   *Opposing*

Step 1, 2, or 3   *Step 4 or 5*
Are the arms noticeably active?   Do both arms move in
                                           opposition to the legs or just
                                           one?

No   *Yes*   *One*   *Both*

Step 1   *Step 2 or 3*   *Step 4*   *Step 5*
Bilateral inactive Do the arms pump up and Semiopposition   Opposing assist
                   down or wing?

Wing   *Pump*

Step 2   *Step 3*
Bilateral reactive Bilateral assist

Only slight arm movement

Arm held out to side

Arm opposite swing leg comes forward with that leg

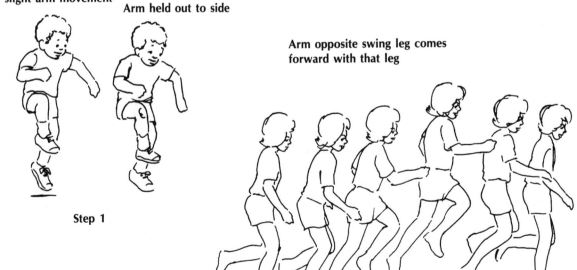

Step 1

Step 4

Name _____ Section _____ Date _____

LABORATORY 8: ASSESSING THE DEVELOPMENTAL LEVEL OF HOPPING

OBSERVATION CHECKLIST: *Hopping*

Observation number	1	2	3	4	5	6	7
Hopper's name							
Hopper's age							
Date							
Observation type[a]							
Component							
Leg action							
Step 1. Momentary flight							
Step 2. Fall and catch; swing leg inactive							
Step 3. Projected takeoff; swing leg assists							
Step 4. Projection delay; swing leg leads							
Arm action							
Step 1. Bilateral inactive							
Step 2. Bilateral reactive							
Step 3. Bilateral assist							
Step 4. Semiopposition							
Step 5. Opposing assist							
Summary profile							
Leg							
Arm							

Note. From *Developing Children—Their Changing Movement* (p. 54) by M.A. Roberton and L.E. Halverson, 1984, Philadelphia, PA: Lea & Febiger. Copyright 1984 by Lea & Febiger. Adapted by permission.

[a]Codes for observation type: D = direct; P = photographs; F = film; V = video; s = slow motion.

Discussion Questions

1. Did you find instances where a performer was at a different level on a subsequent attempt of a skill? If so, describe them.

(Cont.)

2. Did an older child or adult perform at a lower level than someone younger? Describe any such instances.

3. Were any individuals at different levels for different body components? If so, describe.

4. How did your instructions make a difference in skill performance? How might different cue words elicit a more advanced performance level? In what body component(s)?

5. What were the differences among the methods of observation (photos, slow-motion video, etc.)? Which method was the easiest and which the hardest? What are the disadvantages of each observation method in making an accurate assessment?

9

Assessing the Developmental Level of Throwing

Overarm throwing is the most difficult of the basic skill assessments. There are more body components to be observed than in any other skill, and, like in jumping, only one action is performed at a time. Each throw is executed quickly, and viewing from two angles is required for several components.

The best way to prepare for this challenge is to know the developmental steps in Table 4.6 on pages 124 and 125 of your textbook and the observation guide. Additionally, extra study of the illustrations in the textbook will help. You might even want to obtain photos of baseball pitchers to identify some of the important criteria for skilled throwing.

Objectives
- To become familiar with an observation plan for overarm throwing.
- To practice categorizing throwers into developmental levels by practicing with photographs, then videotapes or films, and finally in person.
- To gain enough proficiency to categorize throwers quickly.

Format
Independent work, about 20 minutes; class or free time to watch videotapes or films, about 25 minutes; clinical setting to observe throwers, about 25 minutes.

Textbook Reading
"Overarm Throwing" on pages 121-130

Procedure
1. Using the photographs provided, categorize throwers as you follow the observation plan. Notice that you have more body components to observe for throwing than for the other basic skills. As you make your decisions, check the appropriate boxes on the checklist, then complete the summary profile.

2. If your instructor schedules you to watch a videotape or film, watch several throwers in slow motion if you can. It is best if the filming angle is varied because many decisions are based on observation from a specified location. Finally, categorize several throwers at full-speed viewing.

3. Following your practice with photographs and videotapes, observe throwers in person. Decide beforehand what instructions you will give, particularly where the thrower should stand and the direction of the throw. Young children may have to be instructed to throw overhand. It is important to provide a ball that can be held easily in one hand.

4. As suggested in the jumping laboratory, a change in instructions may change the thrower's quality of movement. For example, you might say "throw harder,"

"throw farther," or "throw faster" to the throwers, then categorize them a second time to see if the result varies.

5. Be ready to defend your categorizations in a class discussion.

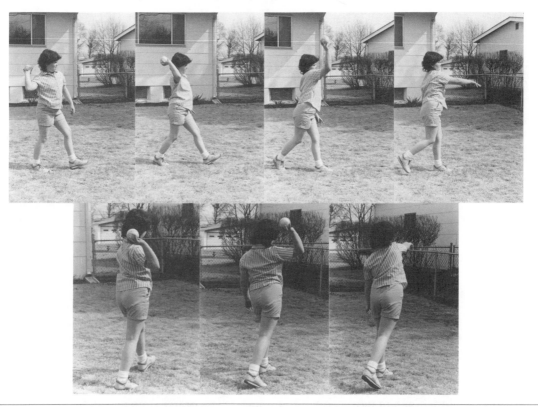

Figure 9.1. CH, age 8.9 years, throwing.

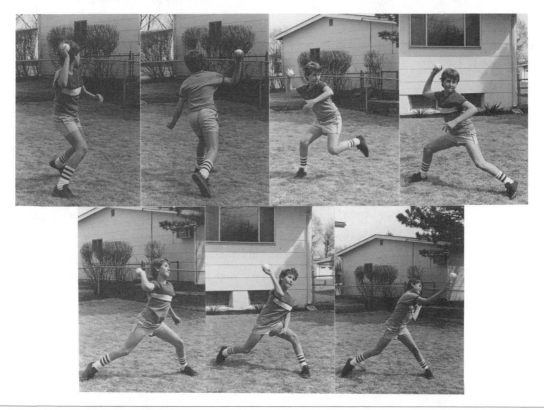

Figure 9.2. MH, age 12.0 years, throwing.

OBSERVATION PLAN FOR THROWING

Foot Action
Watch the feet from the side: Is
a step taken?

No   Yes

Step 1
No step

Step 2, 3, or 4
Is the step homo- or contralateral?

Homo-   Contra-

Step 2
Homolateral step

Step 3 or 4
Is the step over half the
thrower's height?

No   Yes

Step 3
Contralateral, short step

Step 4
Contralateral, long step

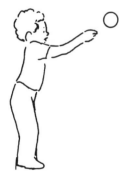

Step 1

Step 3

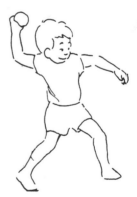

Step 4

Trunk Action
Move to watch the trunk from
the side and the rear: Are there
rotary movements?

No /   \ Yes

Step 1
No trunk action or flexion-
extension

Step 2 or 3
Does the lower trunk (hips)
rotate?

No /   \ Yes

Watch from the rear: Do the
hips start forward before the
trunk?

No /   \ Yes

Step 2
Block or upper trunk rotation

Step 3
Differentiated rotation

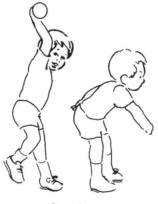

Step 1

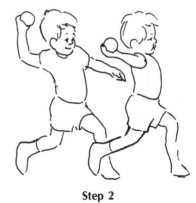

Step 2

Backswing
Watch from the front and side:
Does the arm move backward
before moving forward?

No / Yes

Step 1
No backswing

Does the hand drop below the
waist?

No / Yes

Step 2 or 3
Does the ball swing outward,
up and around?

Step 4
Circular, downward backswing

No / Yes

Step 2
Elbow and humeral flexion

Step 3
Circular upward backswing

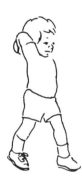

Step 2

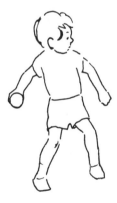

Step 4

Humerus Action
Watch from the side: Do the
elbow and upper arm move forward at shoulder level (humerus
forms a right angle with the
trunk)?

No ⟋   ⟍ *Yes*

Step 1
Humerus oblique

Step 2 or 3
At the moment of front-facing,
is the elbow pointed toward
you at the side, or is it seen
outside the outline of the body?

Outside ⟋   ⟍ *To side*

Step 2
Humerus aligned but independent

Step 3
Humerus lags

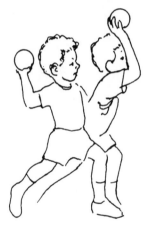

Step 2

Step 3

Forearm
Watch the ball in the thrower's
hand: Does it move forward
steadily or drop downward or
stay stationary as the thrower
rotates forward?

Steadily forward ⟋   ⟍ *Stays stationary / Drops down*

Step 1
No forearm lag

Is the deepest lag reached before or at front-facing? (May be
difficult to see without slow-
motion film or videotape)

Before ⟋   ⟍ *At*

Step 2
Forearm lag

Step 3
Delayed forearm lag

Name _____ **Section** _____ **Date** _____

LABORATORY 9: ASSESSING THE DEVELOPMENTAL LEVEL OF THROWING

OBSERVATION CHECKLIST: *Throwing*

Observation number	1	2	3	4	5	6	7
Thrower's name							
Thrower's age							
Date							
Observation type[a]							
Component							
Foot action							
Step 1. No step							
Step 2. Homolateral							
Step 3. Contralateral, short							
Step 4. Contralateral, long							
Trunk action							
Step 1. None/forward-back							
Step 2. Block/upper trunk only							
Step 3. Differentiated rotation							
Arm Action: backswing							
Step 1. No backswing							
Step 2. Elbow and humeral flexion							
Step 3. Circular, upward							
Step 4. Circular, downward							
Arm action: humerus							
Step 1. Humerus oblique							
Step 2. Humerus aligned, independent							
Step 3. Humerus lags							
Arm action: forearm							
Step 1. No lag							
Step 2. Forearm lag							
Step 3. Delayed lag							

[a]Codes for observation type: D = direct; P = photographs; F = film; V = video; s = slow motion.

(Cont.)

LABORATORY 9 (Cont.)

Observation number	1	2	3	4	5	6	7
Summary profile							
Foot							
Trunk							
Backswing							
Humerus							
Forearm							

Name _____ Section _____ Date _____

Discussion Questions

1. Did you find instances where a performer was at a different level on a subsequent attempt of a skill? If so, describe them.

2. Did an older child or adult perform at a lower level than someone younger? Describe any such instances.

3. Were any individuals at different levels for different body components? If so, describe.

4. How did your instructions make a difference in skill performance? How might different cue words elicit a more advanced performance level? In what body component(s)?

(Cont.)

5. How might the task (for example, throwing fast versus throwing far) or the equipment (for example, the size of the ball) influence the level of performance? What might you change to elicit a more advanced level? State the body component and level involved.

6. What were the differences among the methods of observation (photos, slow-motion video, etc.)? Which method was the easiest and which the hardest? What are the disadvantages of each observation method in making an accurate assessment?

7. If you completed Laboratory 6 or 8, did it take longer to assess repetitive skills such as running and hopping or a discrete skill such as throwing? Why?

10

Assessing the Developmental Level of Sidearm Striking

Recall from your textbook that the leg, trunk, and humerus (upper-arm) actions for sidearm striking are similar to those for throwing. You would have the materials to assess sidearm striking just by adding a developmental sequence for racquet or bat action to the materials in the last laboratory exercise. This laboratory does just that.

If you have worked extensively on overarm throwing assessment, it would be acceptable to observe just racquet or bat action for this exercise. If not, use the observation guides from the overarm throwing laboratory to complete observation of all the body components in sidearm striking. Of course, the more you practice, the better, so you may assess all the body components in either case.

Objectives
- To become familiar with an observation plan for racquet or bat action in sidearm striking.
- To practice categorizing strikers into developmental levels, first with photographs, videotapes, or films, then in person.
- To develop enough proficiency to categorize strikers quickly.

Format
Independent work, about 10 minutes; class or free time to view videotapes or films, about 15 minutes; clinical setting to observe strikers, about 15 minutes.

Textbook Reading
"Sidearm Striking" on pages 132-135

Procedure
1. As with the previous laboratory exercises, categorize the strikers in the photographs as you follow the observation plan. Check the appropriate boxes on the checklist, then complete the summary profile.
2. If your instructor schedules you to view a videotape or film, watch a striker in slow motion if possible. Then categorize several strikers at full-speed viewing.
3. Observe striking in person. You will have to decide beforehand whether to use a stationary ball or to have someone "pitch" to the striker. You will also have to select the size and weight of the racquet or bat according to the size of the performer.
4. Be prepared to defend your categorizations in a class discussion.

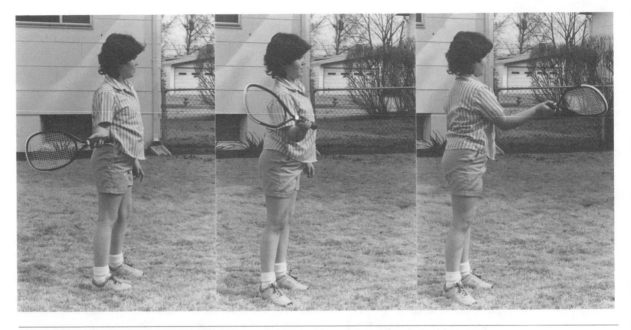

Figure 10.1. CH, age 8.9 years, striking.

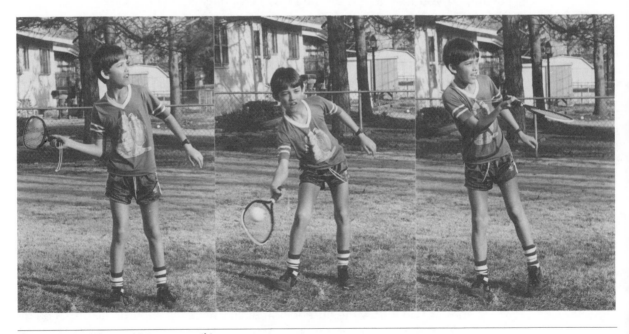

Figure 10.2. KS, age 10.2 years, striking.

OBSERVATION PLAN FOR SIDEARM STRIKING
(for foot, trunk, and humerus components, use the *throwing* observation)

Racquet/Bat Action
Is the racquet swung in a
horizontal plane?

No / Yes

Step 1
Chop

Steps 2 to 4
Does the racquet "lag" (pause
in forward motion)?

No / Yes

Step 2
Arm swing only

Does the racquet "lag" occur at
the "front facing" position?

No / Yes

Step 3
Racquet lag

Step 4
Delayed racquet lag

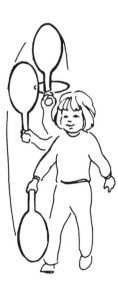

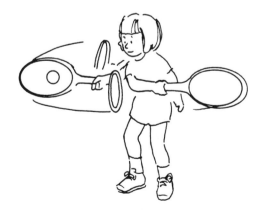

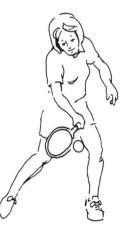

Step 1   Step 2   Step 4

Name _____ Section _____ Date _____

LABORATORY 10: ASSESSING THE DEVELOPMENTAL LEVEL OF SIDEARM STRIKING

OBSERVATION CHECKLIST: *Striking*

Observation number	1	2	3	4	5	6	7
Striker's name							
Striker's age							
Date							
Observation type[a]							
Component							
Racquet/bat action							
Step 1. Chop							
Step 2. Arm swing only							
Step 3. Racquet Lag							
Step 4. Delayed Lag							
Humerus action							
Step 1. Humerus oblique							
Step 2. Aligned, independent							
Step 3. Humerus lags							
Trunk action							
Step 1. None/forward-back							
Step 2. Block/upper trunk							
Step 3. Differentiated rotation							
Foot action							
Step 1. No step							
Step 2. Homolateral							
Step 3. Contralateral, short							
Step 4. Contralateral, long							
Summary profile							
Racquet							
Humerus							
Trunk							
Foot							

[a]Codes for observation type: D = direct; P = photographs; F = film; V = video; s = slow motion.

Name _____ Section _____ Date _____

Discussion Questions

1. Did you find instances where a performer was at a different level on a subsequent attempt of a skill? If so, describe them.

2. Did an older child or adult perform at a lower level than someone younger? Describe any such instances.

3. Were any individuals at different levels for different body components? If so, describe.

(Cont.)

4. How did your instructions make a difference in skill performance? How might different cue words elicit a more advanced performance level? In what body component(s)?

5. How might the task (for example, striking a stationary ball versus a moving ball) or the equipment (for example, the weight of the striking implement) influence the level of performance? What might you change to elicit a more advanced level? State the body component and level involved.

6. What were the differences among the methods of observation (photos, slow-motion video, etc.)? Which method was the easiest and which the hardest? What are the disadvantages of each observation method in making an accurate assessment?

11

Assessing the Developmental Level of Catching

Catching is the last, but not the least, of the basic skills to assess in this series of laboratory activities. Recall that catching development may actually lag behind throwing development for a time in childhood. Hence, it is important for professionals to attend to catching development in children. Selection of the type and size of ball to be caught is critical to the results you obtain in your assessments. In fact, you can vary your activities in this laboratory, compared to previous ones, by assessing one child in a clinical setting with several types of balls and a beanbag, rather than assessing several children.

Objectives
- To assess catching development in children by following an observation guide.
- To observe the influence of varying ball size on the developmental level of catching.

Format
Independent work, about 10 minutes; clinical setting to observe catching, about 10 minutes.

Textbook Reading
"Catching Skills" on pages 135-138

Procedure
1. Use the photographs to follow the observation guide, and categorize the children pictured. Remember it may be difficult to make a judgment about body action from still photographs.
2. In a clinical setting, observe the catching skills of several children (or categorize one child catching several different types and sizes of balls and a beanbag).
3. Be ready to defend your categorizations in a class discussion.

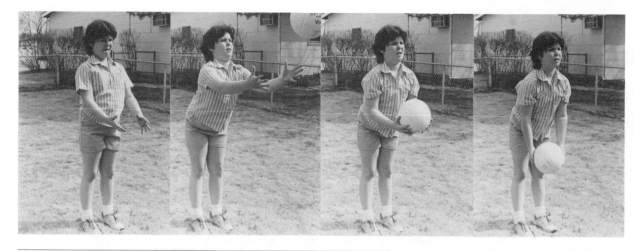

Figure 11.1. CH, age 8.9 years, catching.

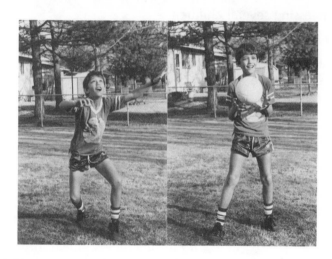

Figure 11.2. KS, age 10.2 years, catching.

OBSERVATION PLAN FOR CATCHING

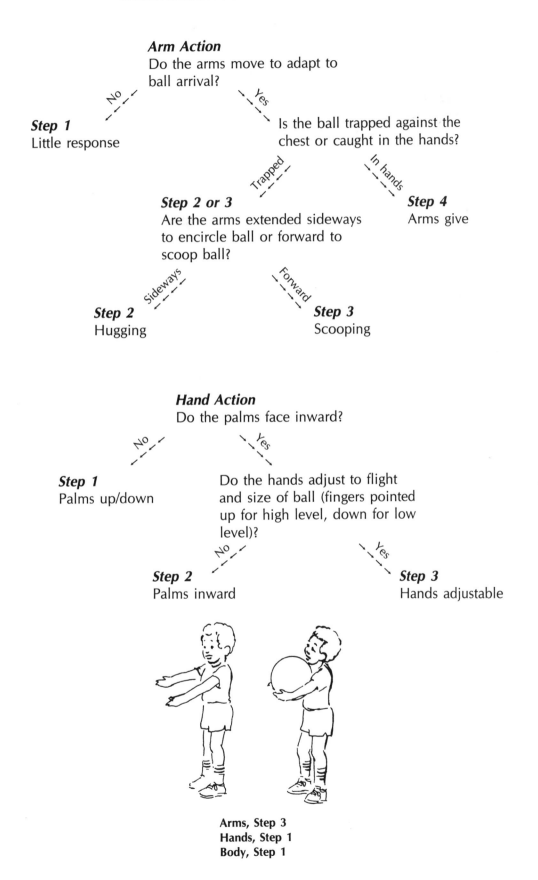

Arm Action
Do the arms move to adapt to
ball arrival?

No / Yes

Step 1
Little response

Is the ball trapped against the
chest or caught in the hands?

Trapped / In hands

Step 2 or 3
Are the arms extended sideways
to encircle ball or forward to
scoop ball?

Step 4
Arms give

Sideways / Forward

Step 2
Hugging

Step 3
Scooping

Hand Action
Do the palms face inward?

No / Yes

Step 1
Palms up/down

Do the hands adjust to flight
and size of ball (fingers pointed
up for high level, down for low
level)?

No / Yes

Step 2
Palms inward

Step 3
Hands adjustable

Arms, Step 3
Hands, Step 1
Body, Step 1

Body Action
Does body move to adjust to
flight of the ball?

No ⟋   Yes ⟍

Step 1
No adjustment

Is body adjustment delayed to
make an accurate movement?

No ⟋   Yes ⟍

Step 2
Premature adjustment

Step 3
Delayed adjustment

Name _____ Section _____ Date _____

LABORATORY 11: ASSESSING THE DEVELOPMENTAL LEVEL OF CATCHING

OBSERVATION CHECKLIST: Catching

Observation number	1	2	3	4	5	6	7
Catcher's name							
Catcher's age							
Date							
Observation type[a]							
Component							
Arm action							
Step 1. Little response							
Step 2. Hugging							
Step 3. Scooping							
Step 4. Arms give							
Hand action							
Step 1. Palms up/down							
Step 2. Palms inward							
Step 3. Hands adjustable							
Body action							
Step 1. No adjustment							
Step 2. Premature adjustment							
Step 3. Delayed adjustment							
Summary profile							
Arm							
Hand							
Body							

[a]Codes for observation type: D = direct; P = photographs; F = film; V = video; s = slow motion.

Discussion Questions

1. Did you find instances where a performer was at a different level on a subsequent attempt of a skill? If so, describe them.

2. Did an older child or adult perform at a lower level than someone younger? Describe any such instances.

3. Were any individuals at different levels for different body components? If so, describe.

4. How might the size or weight of the ball being caught influence the level of performance?

12

Hypothesizing Developmental Sequences

The previous laboratory exercises in assessing skill development should have helped to refine your observation skills. Of course, you were provided with an observation plan, based on developmental sequences identified through research. What happens when you want to assess a skill for which you do not have a developmental sequence? It is possible in this case to hypothesize a developmental sequence from which you could derive an observation plan and checklist. This sequence might not be as refined as one based on research, but it may suit your purpose perfectly well.

In this laboratory you will hypothesize a developmental sequence, an observation guide, and a checklist for kicking, based on readings in the textbook and your knowledge of kicking. Then you can try out your materials!

Objectives
- To experience the process of hypothesizing a developmental sequence.
- To design an observation plan and a checklist from a developmental sequence.
- To refine an observation guide based on use of the guide.

Format
Independent work, about 30 minutes; clinical setting to observe several kickers, about 15 minutes.

Textbook Reading
"Kicking" on pages 130-132

Procedure
1. From what you have read about the developmental changes in kicking, decide which body components will have developmental sequences. Then title and describe two to four developmental steps for each body component on the Developmental Steps for Kicking.

2. Based on your sequences, design an observation plan for each body component and outline it on the Observation Plan for Kicking. Try to design your plan so that one decision is made at any one time. Don't forget to designate the angle from which the observation is made. You might want to include some stick-figure sketches in your plan.

3. On the blank Observation Checklist for Kicking, enter the number and titles of the sequential steps you identified. (Refer to one of the checklists in Laboratories 6 through 11 for a model.)

4. Using the sequential photographs, try out your observation plan. You might find it necessary to refine and revise it. After making any changes you think necessary, try out your revised materials on several kickers.

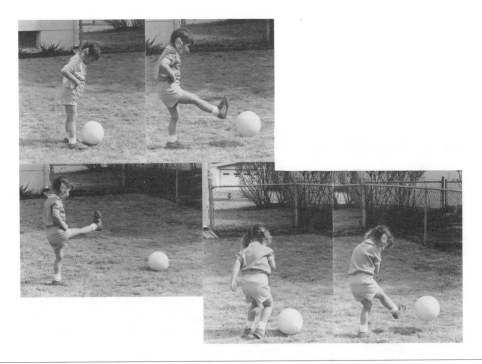

Figure 12.1. LH, age 3.2 years, kicking.

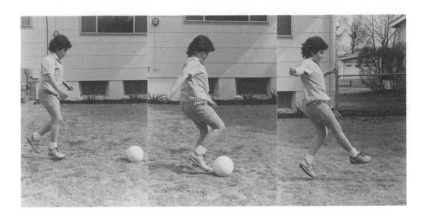

Figure 12.2. CH, age 8.9 years, kicking.

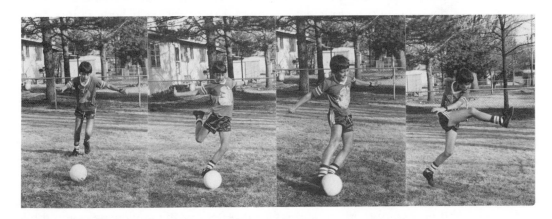

Figure 12.3. KS, age 10.2 years, kicking.

Name _____ Section _____ Date _____

LABORATORY 12: HYPOTHESIZING DEVELOPMENTAL SEQUENCES
Developmental Steps for Kicking

Body Component: _____

Step number	Title	Description

Body Component: _____

Step number	Title	Description

Body Component: _____

Step number	Title	Description

OBSERVATION PLAN FOR KICKING

Component: _____

Component: _____

Component: _____

Name _____ Section _____ Date _____

LABORATORY 12: HYPOTHESIZING DEVELOPMENTAL SEQUENCES

OBSERVATION CHECKLIST: *Kicking*

Observation number	1	2	3	4	5	6	7
Kicker's name							
Kicker's age							
Date							
Observation type[a]							
Component							
_____							
Step _____							
Step _____							
Step _____							
Step _____							
Step _____							
_____							
Step _____							
Step _____							
Step _____							
Step _____							
Step _____							
_____							
Step _____							
Step _____							
Step _____							
Step _____							
Step _____							
Summary profile							
_____							
_____							
_____							

[a]Codes for observation type: D = direct; P = photographs; F = film; V = video; s = slow motion.

Discussion Questions

1. Did you find your initial sequence and observation plan workable? What worked well? What problems did you encounter?

2. Did you revise your initial sequence and observation plan? How? For what other skills might an elementary physical education teacher want to hypothesize a developmental sequence?

PART

IV

Assessing Skills by Quantity and Task Difficulty

There are many systems for assessing motor development. The laboratory activities in Part III used a qualitative assessment. Other assessment systems are discussed in chapter 5 of your textbook. One alternative is to gauge skill development by quantity, that is, by measuring how far, how high, how fast, and so on. Another is to gauge skill by ability to perform increasingly more difficult variations. For example, a child might learn first to hit a ball from a batting tee, then to bat a large plastic ball tossed underhand,

then to hit a baseball thrown overhand. Each method of assessing skill can be appropriate for an individual with a certain degree of skill, for a specified purpose, in a particular setting.

In laboratory activities 13 and 14 you will work with a quantitative system for measuring motor development and a task analysis. The first involves running speed and distance jumped. The second will give you experience in varying task difficulty.

13

Measuring Quantitative Improvement

Quantitative assessment is particularly useful once performers have reached higher levels of qualitative development. For example, a child might have very good running form; further assessments of running ability would typically be measurements of speed. In this laboratory activity you will be summarizing and analyzing two quantitative measurements collected by the physical education teachers at an elementary school in St. Louis County, Missouri, over a two-year period. These scores can be examined for improvement as the children grew and for gender differences.

Objectives
- To summarize the scores of a group of children on running the 50-yard dash and the standing long jump.
- To plot children's quantitative scores over a two-year period.
- To examine quantitative scores for improvement trends and gender differences.

Format   Independent work

Textbook Reading   "Quantitative Improvement in Motor Performance" on pages 142-151

Procedure
1. Calculate the group average for each sex on the dash for each time the students were measured (at ages 8.0, 8.5, 9.0, and 9.5) by dividing the sum of the scores by the number of students.
2. Calculate the combined group average by adding the males' sum to the females' sum and dividing this total sum by the total number of students.
3. Calculate the average yards per second. Divide 50 yards by the average number of seconds taken by the boys, by the girls, and by the combined group at each age.
4. Graph these scores on the grid provided. Use different colors and types of lines (solid, dashed, etc.) to plot the boys' scores, the girls' scores, and the combined group scores. Be sure to label the axes.
5. Repeat the same calculations for the standing long jump scores and graph the standing long jump scores in the same manner as the dash scores.

Name _____ Section _____ Date _____

LABORATORY 13: MEASURING QUANTITATIVE IMPROVEMENT
Data Sheet: 50-Yard Dash Performance in Seconds

	Time 1 Age 8.0	Time 2 Age 8.5	Time 3 Age 9.0	Time 4 Age 9.5
Boys				
Student 1	7.9 (70)[a]	8.2 (50)	8.4 (45)	8.1 (55)
Student 2	9.1 (16)	8.8 (30)	8.8 (30)	7.9 (70)
Student 3	7.8 (80)	7.8 (80)	7.7 (85)	7.2 (96)
Student 4	8.7 (35)	9.3 (12)	8.4 (45)	8.1 (55)
Student 5	8.4 (45)	8.0 (65)	7.7 (85)	7.8 (80)
Student 6	9.0 (20)	9.3 (12)	7.8 (80)	8.8 (30)
Student 7	8.9 (25)	8.8 (30)	8.0 (65)	8.2 (50)
Total	_____	_____	_____	_____
Average	_____	_____	_____	_____
Yards per second	_____	_____	_____	_____
Girls				
Student 1	10.7 (03)	9.5 (17)	9.1 (25)	8.8 (45)
Student 2	8.6 (50)	8.0 (80)	8.4 (60)	8.3 (65)
Student 3	9.4 (20)	8.8 (45)	8.5 (55)	8.3 (65)
Student 4	10.0 (08)	10.0 (08)	8.2 (67)	8.2 (67)
Student 5	8.5 (55)	7.9 (82)	7.7 (86)	7.7 (86)
Student 6	8.7 (47)	7.8 (85)	7.9 (82)	7.9 (82)
Student 7	8.3 (65)	8.1 (70)	7.8 (85)	7.7 (86)
Total	_____	_____	_____	_____
Average	_____	_____	_____	_____
Yards per second	_____	_____	_____	_____
Combined group total	_____	_____	_____	_____
Combined group average	_____	_____	_____	_____
Combined yards per second	_____	_____	_____	_____

[a]Numbers in parentheses are the percentile scores associated with raw scores for this age as reported in the AAHPER Fitness Test Manual.

50-YARD DASH SCORES

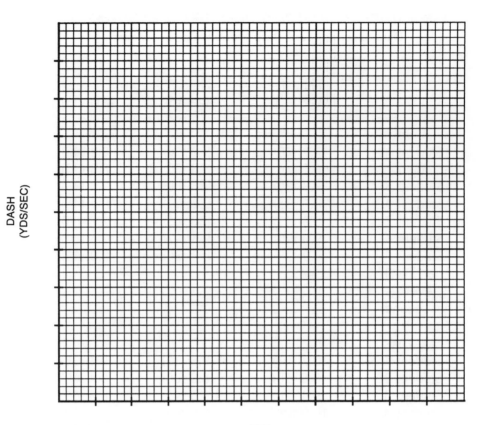

DASH
(YDS/SEC)

AGE

Name _____ Section _____ Date _____

Data Sheet: Standing Long Jump Performance in Inches

	Time 1 Age 8.0	Time 2 Age 8.5	Time 3 Age 9.0	Time 4 Age 9.5
Boys				
Student 1	64 (75)[a]	66 (80)	63 (70)	66 (80)
Student 2	50 (15)	54 (25)	59 (50)	61 (65)
Student 3	60 (55)	66 (80)	72 (95)	72 (95)
Student 4	50 (15)	54 (25)	55 (30)	56 (35)
Student 5	54 (25)	54 (25)	57 (40)	57 (40)
Student 6	43 (02)	51 (16)	51 (16)	51 (16)
Student 7	48 (10)	56 (35)	48 (10)	59 (50)
Total	_____	_____	_____	_____
Average	_____	_____	_____	_____
Girls				
Student 1	39 (04)	47 (15)	50 (27)	46 (12)
Student 2	54 (40)	59 (62)	61 (72)	59 (62)
Student 3	52 (32)	51 (30)	55 (45)	60 (70)
Student 4	61 (72)	61 (72)	63 (81)	58 (60)
Student 5	51 (30)	59 (62)	60 (70)	57 (55)
Student 6	63 (81)	61 (72)	72 (94)	72 (94)
Student 7	60 (70)	62 (80)	71 (94)	66 (86)
Total	_____	_____	_____	_____
Average	_____	_____	_____	_____
Combined group total	_____	_____	_____	_____
Combined group average	_____	_____	_____	_____

[a]Numbers in parentheses are the percentile scores associated with raw scores for this age as reported in the AAHPER Fitness Test Manual.

STANDING LONG JUMP SCORES

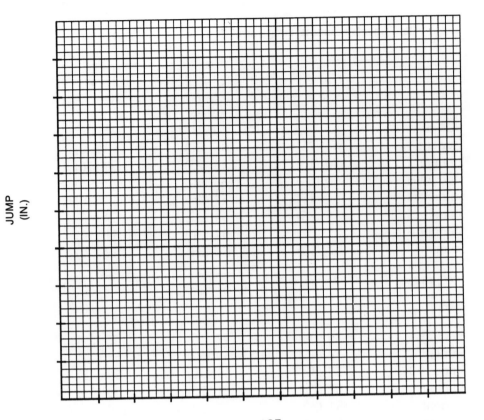

JUMP
(IN.)

AGE

Name _____ Section _____ Date _____

Discussion Questions

1. Did the students improve with age? What changes in physical growth might have contributed to improved scores? What qualitative skill improvements might have contributed to quantitative improvements? How would you explain any lack of improvement?

2. Compare the shape of your graphs to those in Figures 5.1 and 5.3 (pages 143 and 145) of your textbook at similar ages. Are the shapes similar? Is this what you expected? Why or why not?

(Cont.)

3. Compare the actual scores (the number of yards per second running and the inches jumped) to Figures 5.1 and 5.3 (pages 143 and 145) of your textbook. Are they similar? What might account for any differences?

4. Did you find the same gender differences in these students as reflected in Figures 5.1 through 5.4 in your textbook? Explain.

5. Look at the percentile scores of the students, which are in parentheses after the raw scores on the data sheets. How do these students generally compare to national norms?

14

Tracking Skill Refinement Through Task Analyses

Qualitative and quantitative change are not the only components of motor development. Skill development also involves an improving ability to adapt performance to varying environmental situations, to execute increasingly more difficult skills. For example, being able to kick a soccer ball into a goal is desirable, but using kicking skill in a game will demand adaptations for varying locations, distances, goalie and defensive player positions, and so on. For a teacher or coach to gauge task difficulty, a system of classification is necessary. Task analysis is one method of classifying skill tasks. Teachers can use it both to assess their students as they refine their skills and to plan appropriate practice activities. A task analysis allows identification of a progressively more challenging task as performers become proficient at a simpler one.

A task analysis is conducted by identifying the factors involved and rating levels of these factors from simple to complex. Several examples of a task analysis are given in Figures 5.7 and 5.8 on pages 154 and 155 of the textbook. You will practice analyzing kicking in this laboratory activity.

Objectives
- To learn a system for classifying skill tasks by level of difficulty.
- To become familiar with factors that influence task difficulty and how levels of these factors can vary from simple to complex.
- To practice structuring a game or drill at a specified level of difficulty using a task analysis model.

Format Independent work

Textbook Reading "Skill Refinement" on pages 153-156

Procedure
1. On the Kicking Activity Chart, fill in levels of difficulty from simple to complex for each factor listed across the top of the chart.
2. Using a dotted line, connect the level in each column that would result in a simple kicking task. See Figure 5.7 (page 154) in your textbook for an example.
3. Using a solid line, do the same for levels that would result in a complex kicking task.

Name _____ Section _____ Date _____

Kicking Activity Chart

F A C T O R S	Size of object being kicked	Weight of object being kicked	Distance object must be kicked	Accuracy required of kick	Trajectory required of kick	Movement of the object being kicked	Spatial adjustments required of body	Movement characteristics of the target
S I M P L E L E V E L S T O C O M P L E X								

Note. From "Developmental Task Analysis: The Design of Movement Experiences and Evaluation of Motor Development Status" by J. Herkowitz, 1978, in *Motor Development* by M.V. Ridenour (Ed.), Princeton, NJ: Princeton Book Company. Copyright 1978 by M.V. Ridenour. Adapted by permission of J. Herkowitz and M.V. Ridenour.

Discussion Questions

1. Describe an activity, drill, or game you could conduct with elementary school children that incorporates the simple kicking task you identified on the chart.

2. Describe an activity, drill, or game you could conduct with high school students that incorporates the complex task you identified on the chart.

PART

V

Assessing Correlates of Motor Development

Part II of your textbook surveys various factors that affect motor development, including perceptual change, physiological change, cognitive change, and sociocultural practices. In this section you will have the opportunity to work with aspects of these correlative factors. Your instructor will assign some or all of these laboratory activities as experience dictates and time allows.

In some cases, other courses in your program of study will take you beyond the laboratory activity outlined here. Your instructor may determine that time is best spent elsewhere. Any of these laboratory activities will give you an opportunity to examine aspects of motor development more closely and to relate your observations to your readings.

15

Testing Perceptual-Motor Development

Chapter 6 in your textbook recounts the controversy over the relationship between perceptual-motor and cognitive deficiencies. At the same time, the value of testing perceptual-motor development was recognized as a necessary means of identifying children with perceptual-motor deficiencies. Children with such deficiencies then could be given remedial activities to improve their perceptual-motor skills.

The published perceptual-motor surveys vary in content, often reflecting the emphasis favored by the author. That is, one survey might have many items testing visual perception, another sensory integration, and so on. The survey in this laboratory was designed to familiarize you with some common ways to test visual, kinesthetic, and auditory perception. It does not have established reliability or validity, but it will show you how perceptual-motor development is tested.

Objectives
- To become familiar with perceptual-motor test items.
- To observe a child's performance on perceptual-motor tasks.

Format   Clinical setting, about 20 minutes

Textbook Readings   "Visual Development," "Kinesthetic Development," and "Auditory Development" on pages 170-186 and "Kephart's Theory" on pages 191-195

Equipment Needed
- Pencil
- Low balance beam
- Three blocks of the same size but different colors
- Small jingle bell
- *Life Span Motor Development*

Procedure
1. Give the test items on the survey to a child between 5 and 7 years of age. Your instructor may arrange for you to visit a school or program, or you will be asked to locate a young child on your own.
2. Obtain the child's birthdate and calculate a decimal age. Ask the child to write his or her name to determine the dominant hand. Record this information on the data sheet.
3. Conduct the tests for visual, kinesthetic, and auditory perception according to the directions given at the beginning of each test. Before conducting each test, briefly explain it to the child. Record your results in the spaces provided.

Name _____ Section _____ Date _____

LABORATORY 15: TESTING PERCEPTUAL-MOTOR DEVELOPMENT
Survey and Data Sheet

Child writes first name _____

Sex _____ Birthdate _____ Decimal age _____ Dominant hand   R   L

I. Visual Perception: Size Constancy and Spatial Orientation

Arrange three blocks on a long table, about three feet from the child, so that they are spread out away from the child, about six inches apart. After the first four questions bring the blocks in front of the child. Ask the questions or give the directions listed below, and record whether or not the response was correct.

Question/Direction	Correct	Incorrect
1. What color is this? (Proceed to others.)	_____	_____
2. Which block is closest to you?	_____	_____
3. Which block is the farthest away?	_____	_____
4. Are the blocks the same size?	_____	_____
5. Place the blocks so that the blue block is higher than the yellow block.	_____	_____
6. Place the blue block so that it is lower than the yellow block but higher than the red block.	_____	_____
Number correct	_____/6	

II. Visual Perception: Whole and Parts

Using the pictures in Figure 6.4 of your textbook, point to one. Ask the child what the picture shows. Record whether the child describes the parts (fruit, candy, etc.), describes the whole picture (a face), or both (a scooter made out of candy). Point to a second picture, and repeat the questions. Record the category of response.

1. _____ Parts   _____ Whole   _____ Both
2. _____ Parts   _____ Whole   _____ Both

III. Kinesthetic Perception: Identification of Body Parts

Give the directions listed, and record whether the child touches the correct or incorrect body part.

Direction	Correct	Incorrect
1. Touch your nose.	_____	_____
2. Touch your hips.	_____	_____
3. Touch your wrists.	_____	_____
4. Touch your knees.	_____	_____
5. Touch your heels.	_____	_____
6. Touch your ears.	_____	_____
7. Touch your shoulders.	_____	_____
Number correct	_____/7	

(Cont.)

LABORATORY 15 (Cont.)

IV. **Kinesthetic Perception: Left/Right Discrimination**

Give the directions listed, and record whether the response is correct or incorrect.

Direction	Correct	Incorrect
1. Touch your right ear.	_____	_____
2. Touch your left knee.	_____	_____
3. Pick up this pencil with your left hand.	_____	_____
4. Is the pencil on your right or left? (Place on right.)	_____	_____
5. Touch your left hip with your right hand.	_____	_____
Number correct	__/5	

V. **Kinesthetic Perception: Balance**

Position the child at one end of a low balance beam, with both feet on the beam. Ask the child to walk along the beam to the other end without falling off. Record the number of steps the child takes before stepping off the beam and whether the beam walk was completed.

Number of steps _____   Walk completed? _____ Yes _____ No

VI. **Auditory Perception: Location**

Holding a small jingle bell, face the child and place both hands behind your back. Place the bell in one and form a fist with each hand to conceal the bell's location. Bring your hands to the front and shake them to make the bell jingle. Ask the child to point to the hand holding the bell. Repeat five times, randomly placing the bell in either hand.

	Correct	Incorrect
1.	_____	_____
2.	_____	_____
3.	_____	_____
4.	_____	_____
5.	_____	_____
Number correct	__/5	

Name _____ Section _____ Date _____

Discussion Questions

1. Which aspects of perceptual-motor development seemed to be well developed in the child with whom you worked? Which perceptual-motor discriminations must yet be refined? Cite results to support your answer.

2. Did vision, kinesthesis, and audition seem to be equally developed? On what do you base your answer?

(Cont.)

3. Using the age ranges for perceptual development mentioned in your textbook, do your results seem appropriate for the age of the child you observed? Why or why not?

4. Were any test items difficult to explain to the child or to score? Would you change any of the test items? If so, how? If not, why?

16

Examining the Development of Cardiovascular Endurance

As discussed in the textbook, physical fitness is multifaceted, and endurance is one fitness component. Endurance for vigorous activity, or working capacity, increases with physical growth as well as training. It is interesting to examine the development of endurance over time, as children are growing. We would expect improved endurance as children grow older and bigger. Since growth spurts for boys and girls occur at different ages, we would expect to see gender differences in endurance development.

In this laboratory exercise you will summarize and analyze the endurance performance of a group of children over a two-year period. Time on the mile run will serve as the measure of endurance. You will use scores actually attained by children in physical education classes at a St. Louis County, Missouri, school.

Objectives
- To examine children's endurance performance scores for improvement with advancing age.
- To identify any gender differences in endurance development at ages eight and nine.

Format   Independent work

Textbook Reading   "Physiological Changes and Exercise" on pages 203-218

Procedure
1. Obtain the average score for the boys at each age tested by summing the scores in each column and dividing by the number of boys.
2. Do the same for the girls.
3. Obtain an average for the combined group by summing the two group totals and dividing by the number of students in the combined group.
4. Graph your average scores on the sheet provided. Graph the boys, the girls, and the combined group scores in different colors or with different types of lines. Remember to label the axes.

Name _____ Section _____ Date _____

LABORATORY 16: EXAMINING THE DEVELOPMENT OF CARDIOVASCULAR ENDURANCE
Data Sheet: Mile-Run Times (in Minutes)

	Time 1 Age 8.0	Time 2 Age 8.5	Time 3 Age 9.0	Time 4 Age 9.5
Boys				
Student 1	8.4 (64)[a]	8.3 (66)	8.4 (63)	8.9 (54)
Student 2	8.8 (57)	8.8 (56)	9.7 (37)	9.7 (37)
Student 3	7.8 (75)	7.3 (81)	7.5 (79)	7.6 (77)
Student 4	11.3 (12)	10.3 (27)	11.0 (16)	9.5 (40)
Student 5	8.8 (57)	8.2 (68)	8.5 (62)	8.6 (60)
Student 6	9.1 (50)	9.7 (37)	8.6 (60)	8.5 (62)
Student 7	13.0 (02)	11.3 (12)	10.4 (25)	10.1 (30)
Total	_____	_____	_____	_____
Average	_____	_____	_____	_____
Girls				
Student 1	11.8 (23)	15.7 (00)	10.0 (60)	11.4 (30)
Student 2	9.3 (74)	8.8 (81)	8.7 (83)	7.9 (91)
Student 3	9.6 (68)	10.0 (61)	9.1 (77)	9.1 (76)
Student 4	15.5 (00)	15.5 (00)	10.6 (46)	9.0 (80)
Student 5	11.8 (23)	11.1 (34)	10.5 (48)	10.1 (56)
Student 6	10.2 (55)	8.8 (82)	9.0 (79)	7.7 (92)
Total	_____	_____	_____	_____
Average	_____	_____	_____	_____
Combined group total	_____	_____	_____	_____
Combined group average	_____	_____	_____	_____

[a]Numbers in parentheses are the percentile scores associated with the raw score for 9- to 10-year-olds on the AAHPER Youth Fitness Test.

CARDIOVASCULAR ENDURANCE SCORES

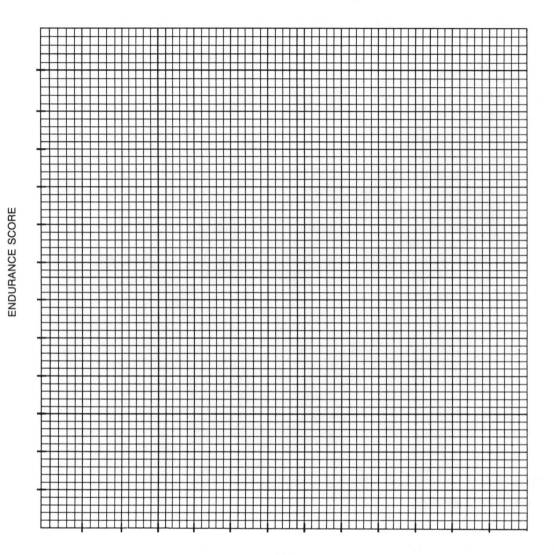

AGE

Name _____ **Section** _____ **Date** _____

Discussion Questions

1. Did endurance scores in the combined group improve as children aged? Were the results as you expected? What did you expect? How did the group perform? If your results were not as expected, how might you account for the discrepancy?

2. Compare the boys' and girls' averages. Did both groups improve with age? After reading the textbook, was this what you expected? Why or why not? How do the absolute scores of the boys and girls compare? Examine the associated percentile scores in parentheses following the raw scores. What does this tell us about the performance of the boys and the girls at this school compared to national norms?

(Cont.)

3. What physical growth measurements would be helpful in assessing whether an individual's performance is consistent with his or her physical maturation? If you were a physical education teacher, how would you use these growth measurements to adjust the goals you set for your students?

4. Did each child improve with age? Describe one who did not, if there was one. What might account for this lack of improvement?

17

Examining Trends in Strength Development

Although strength tends to increase as muscle mass increases with growth, the two are not necessarily parallel. The peak increase in strength typically lags behind the peak increase in muscle mass. We expect strength to increase with growth, but stronger children at a younger age are not always stronger at an older age. Children at a given chronological age are at various levels of physical maturation, therefore differing in muscle mass gain. Too, strength is influenced by training.

It is interesting to observe increases in strength as children grow and to note whether any of the children who are weaker at a young age gain on their peers. In this laboratory activity, you will analyze several strength measurements taken on the same children who provided the scores for the previous laboratory. Functional strength measurements are used: pull-ups (boys), flexed-arm hangs (girls), and sit-ups. Because sit-ups are a functional measurement of abdominal strength and pull-ups and flexed-arm hangs are measurements of arm and shoulder strength, you can compare relative strength in two body areas.

Objectives
- To observe changes in functional strength in children over a two-year time period.
- To examine stability of strength performance in a group of children.
- To identify any gender differences in strength development.
- To examine differential strength development over two body areas.

Format   Independent work

Textbook Reading   "Strength Development" on pages 219-225

Procedure
1. Obtain the average scores for boys on pull-ups at each age by summing their scores and dividing by the number of boys.
2. Do the same for the girls on the flexed-arm hang.
3. Obtain an average sit-up score for the boys, the girls, and the combined group by summing the boys' and girls' totals, then dividing by the total number of students.
4. Graph your average scores on the grid provided. Graph boys', girls', and combined group scores where possible with different colors or different types of lines. Remember to label the axes.

Name _____ Section _____ Date _____

LABORATORY 17: EXAMINING TRENDS IN STRENGTH DEVELOPMENT
Data Sheet: Number of Pull-Ups Performed by Boys

	Time 1 Age 8.0	Time 2 Age 8.5	Time 3 Age 9.0	Time 4 Age 9.5
Student 1	8 (92)	6 (87)	7 (90)	10 (95)
Student 2	4 (80)	3 (75)	3 (75)	5 (85)
Student 3	7 (90)	5 (85)	5 (85)	5 (85)
Student 4	3 (75)	4 (80)	6 (87)	5 (85)
Total	_____	_____	_____	_____
Average	_____	_____	_____	_____

Data Sheet: Flexed-Arm Hang Time (in Seconds) Achieved by Girls

	Time 1 Age 8.0	Time 2 Age 8.5	Time 3 Age 9.0	Time 4 Age 9.5
Student 1	1 (15)	1 (15)	4 (30)	1 (15)
Student 2	5 (35)	3 (25)	16 (70)	26 (86)
Student 3	1 (15)	2 (20)	1 (15)	6 (40)
Student 4	8 (47)	12 (60)	10 (55)	38 (92)
Student 5	11 (57)	9 (50)	11 (57)	5 (35)
Student 6	27 (87)	38 (92)	24 (85)	31 (90)
Student 7	51 (95)	34 (91)	50 (95)	38 (92)
Total	_____	_____	_____	_____
Average	_____	_____	_____	_____

ARM AND SHOULDER STRENGTH SCORES

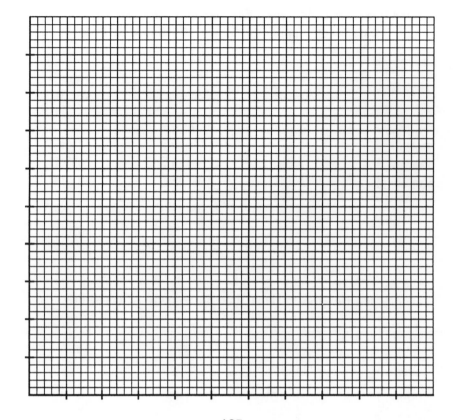

PULL-UPS

ARM HANG

AGE

Name _____ Section _____ Date _____

Data Sheet: Number of Sit-Ups Performed in Sixty Seconds

	Time 1 Age 8.0	Time 2 Age 8.5	Time 3 Age 9.0	Time 4 Age 9.5
Boys				
Student 1	38 (75)	38 (75)	42 (85)	44 (90)
Student 2	35 (60)	21 (15)	26 (27)	29 (40)
Student 3	46 (92)	61 (97)	49 (94)	42 (85)
Student 4	28 (35)	39 (77)	30 (47)	33 (65)
Student 5	29 (40)	59 (97)	48 (94)	30 (45)
Student 6	14 (05)	13 (05)	30 (45)	44 (90)
Student 7	14 (05)	33 (55)	26 (27)	22 (17)
Total	_____	_____	_____	_____
Average	_____	_____	_____	_____
Girls				
Student 1	23 (35)	26 (47)	19 (17)	28 (52)
Student 2	34 (75)	44 (93)	42 (91)	45 (95)
Student 3	19 (17)	39 (87)	37 (82)	36 (81)
Student 4	30 (60)	30 (60)	52 (97)	52 (97)
Student 5	26 (47)	37 (82)	36 (81)	44 (93)
Student 6	25 (45)	30 (60)	35 (80)	38 (85)
Student 7	25 (45)	37 (82)	48 (95)	60 (100)
Total	_____	_____	_____	_____
Average	_____	_____	_____	_____
Combined group total	_____	_____	_____	_____
Combined group average	_____	_____	_____	_____

ABDOMINAL STRENGTH SCORES

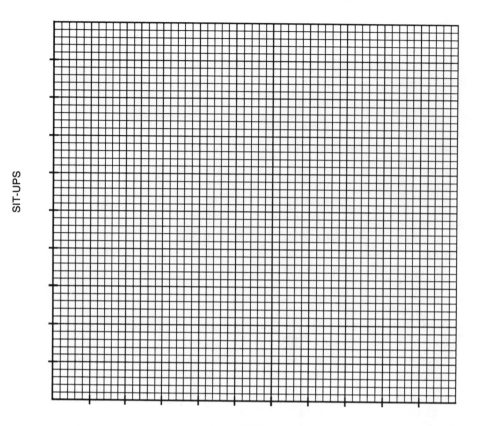

SIT-UPS

AGE

Name _____ **Section** _____ **Date** _____

Discussion Questions

1. Did your subjects get stronger with age? Is this what you expected from the discussion of strength in your textbook? Why?

2. How did the boys and girls compare on sit-ups? Explain this result.

3. Examine the percentile scores in parentheses following the raw scores. Are the students in this group relatively higher in arm strength or abdominal strength? Suggest several reasons for this.

(Cont.)

4. Examine the scores of girl #2 and girl #3. How did their standings in the group change over the two-year period? Examine the scores of boy #3 and boy #5. How did their standings within the group change?

5. Are children with the strongest abdominal strength scores always strongest in arm and shoulder strength? Cite examples to defend your answer.

6. Different tests are used to measure arm strength in boys and girls. What does this tell you about both arm strength differences and growth differences between males and females? How would an increase in fat weight affect performance on these particular measurements? Would boys or girls be more likely to add fat weight over this age period?

18

Assessing Flexibility in Older Adulthood

Range of movement in the joints—flexibility—is determined by elasticity of the body tissues. Unfortunately, inactivity works against elasticity. Most people aren't aware of gradually losing this elasticity until they suddenly realize in middle or late adulthood that they can't move the way they once could. Without a systematic exercise program to maintain and promote flexibility, range of motion begins to shrink in childhood and continues to do so over one's life span.

You will have the opportunity in this laboratory to check the flexibility of a middle-aged or older adult. You will use several simple tests that should not leave your subject sore or stiff. Answers of "No" on the test items indicate the individual has lost flexibility to an extent that affects body function.

Objectives
- To observe the flexibility of a middle-aged or older adult.
- To relate extent of flexibility to extent of physical activity.

Format   Laboratory or clinical setting, about 20 minutes

Textbook Reading   "Development of Flexibility" on pages 227-230

Procedure
1. Practice doing the flexibility tests listed on the data sheet, preferably in front of a mirror.
2. Select an adult over age 50 to perform the flexibility tests as directed on the data sheet. Record your results. Your instructor might arrange for adults to come to your laboratory session, you could visit an adult program, or you may locate an individual on your own.
3. Ask about any exercise programs in which the individual participates, as well as any sport or dance activities done regularly or tasks at home or work that are physical (e.g., gardening). Make notes on the interview on the bottom of your data sheet.

Name _____ Section _____ Date _____

LABORATORY 18: ASSESSING FLEXIBILITY IN OLDER ADULTHOOD
Data Sheet

Subject's sex _____ Subject's birthdate _____ Subject's age _____

Test	Result
1. Have your subject sit on the floor with the back against a wall. Direct the subject to stretch one leg out in front, then draw the foot of the other leg up against the thigh. Is the knee of the extended leg flat against the floor?	____ Yes ____ No
2. Direct your subject to raise arms overhead, fingertips pointing to the ceiling. Are the arms even with or behind the ears?	____ Yes ____ No
Are the arms equally flexible?	____ Yes ____ No
3. Have your subject stand facing you, arms at sides. Direct the subject to turn hands outward without moving the elbows away from the body. Can you see the palms?	____ Yes ____ No
Are the palms equally visible?	____ Yes ____ No
4. Direct your subject to stand, to place arms behind the back and link hands; then pull the hands away from the back. Are the hands raised to a level even with the waist?	____ Yes ____ No

Note. Assessments based on "The Rejuvenation Strategy" by R. Cailliet and L. Gross, 1987, Garden City, NY. Copyright 1987 by Doubleday & Company.

Discussion Questions

1. Has your subject lost flexibility to an extent that body function is affected? Cite results to support your answer. Does this agree with the activity level your subject reported?

(Cont.)

2. Did your subject pass or fail the four tests? Flexibility can vary from joint to joint in an individual: Did you find this to be the case with your subject? Do your results match up with the activities reported by your subject; that is, did she or he report an activity that involves a body area that your test showed had good flexibility?

3. Was your subject equally flexible in the right and left arms and shoulders? What would you have expected based on the textbook discussion? Did your subject report any activity that would account for equal or unequal flexibility?

19

Examining Memory Processing Speed Over the Life Span

The speed with which memory functions are performed varies over the life span. Children take longer than young adults to process information to be remembered. It has been suggested that older adults' memory deficits are due to slowing. In this laboratory exercise you will search for evidence that a trend exists toward faster memory processing speed from childhood to young adulthood, followed by a slowing of memory processing speed in older adulthood.

To examine memory processing speed you will use an experimental paradigm similar to that of Gallagher and Thomas (1980), as described in the textbook on page 251. It is common in skill learning for the learner to perform a practice try, to receive some information about that performance from an instructor, and then to repeat the practice. Such information is termed *knowledge of results* (KR). The time between skill execution and receipt of KR by the learner is the *pre-KR interval*, and between KR and the subsequent skill execution is the *post-KR interval*. Varying the post-KR interval affects skill performance. If the post-KR interval is short, individuals who need more processing time (because their speed of processing is slow) may be greatly affected.

You will use this paradigm to test members of your class, 7-year-olds, and older adults at post-KR intervals of 3 and 12 seconds. Performance might be similar with the longer post-KR interval, but could differ with the shorter interval if any of the age groups requires more processing time. The pre-KR interval will be varied to keep the total time between movements constant.

Objective
- To observe the effect of a shortened post-KR interval on memory processing speed in three age groups.

Format
Laboratory, with a partner, about 1 hour

Textbook Readings
"Speed of Memory Functions" and "Changes in Memory During Older Adulthood" on pages 250-254

Equipment Needed
- A linear slide apparatus or a curvilinear kinesthesiometer (Lafayette 16014)
- A stopwatch or other timing device
- A blindfold

Procedure 1. Select a classmate for a partner. Follow the instructions below to test each other, two 7-year-olds, and two older adults (over age 65). Explain the task to your subjects beforehand.

2. Testing instructions:
    a. Seat the subject before the apparatus and position the blindfold.
    b. Start the timing device.
    c. Instruct the subject to move the number of degrees (with a curvilinear instrument) or centimeters (with a linear slide) stipulated on the data sheet.
    d. Wait the required time interval (12 or 3 seconds), then give KR by saying, "You moved _____ degrees/centimeters." Record this result.
    e. Again wait the required time interval (3 or 12 seconds), then administer the next trial.
    f. Finish one column of trials, then administer the other column, changing the pre- and post-KR intervals.

3. With each pair of subjects, begin one with the long pre-KR/short post-KR set of trials and the other with the short pre-KR/long post-KR set of trials. This balances out any tendency to perform better on the second set of trials because of practice in the first set.

4. Calculate each subject's average error in degrees or centimeters for each set of trials, and contribute your data for the class data sheet. Note that the first trial is not counted because the subject had not yet received KR.

5. Plot your results on the graph provided, using a solid line to connect the 3-second post-KR averages and a dotted line to connect the 12-second post-KR averages.

Name _____ Section _____ Date _____

LABORATORY 19: EXAMINING MEMORY PROCESSING SPEED OVER THE LIFE SPAN
Data Sheet: You and Your Partner

Subject(s) #1 Age: _____ years

Begin with this column:

12-second pre-KR 3-second post-KR			3-second pre-KR 12-second post-KR		
Direct to move	Degrees or cm moved	Error	Direct to move	Degrees or cm moved	Error
80° or 60 cm	_____	XXX	80° or 60 cm	_____	XXX
60° or 45 cm	_____	_____	60° or 45 cm	_____	_____
40° or 30 cm	_____	_____	40° or 30 cm	_____	_____
60° or 45 cm	_____	_____	60° or 45 cm	_____	_____
40° or 30 cm	_____	_____	40° or 30 cm	_____	_____
80° or 60 cm	_____	_____	80° or 60 cm	_____	_____
80° or 60 cm	_____	_____	80° or 60 cm	_____	_____
40° or 30 cm	_____	_____	40° or 30 cm	_____	_____
60° or 45 cm	_____	_____	60° or 45 cm	_____	_____
80° or 60 cm	_____	_____	80° or 60 cm	_____	_____
Total error		_____	Total error		_____
Average error		_____	Average error		_____

Subject(s) #2 Age: _____ years

12-second pre-KR
 3-second post-KR

Begin with this column:

 3-second pre-KR
12-second post-KR

Direct to move	Degrees or cm moved	Error	Direct to move	Degrees or cm moved	Error
80° or 60 cm	_____	XXX	80° or 60 cm	_____	XXX
60° or 45 cm	_____	_____	60° or 45 cm	_____	_____
40° or 30 cm	_____	_____	40° or 30 cm	_____	_____
60° or 45 cm	_____	_____	60° or 45 cm	_____	_____
40° or 30 cm	_____	_____	40° or 30 cm	_____	_____
80° or 60 cm	_____	_____	80° or 60 cm	_____	_____
80° or 60 cm	_____	_____	80° or 60 cm	_____	_____
40° or 30 cm	_____	_____	40° or 30 cm	_____	_____
60° or 45 cm	_____	_____	60° or 45 cm	_____	_____
80° or 60 cm	_____	_____	80° or 60 cm	_____	_____
Total error		_____	Total error		_____
Average error		_____	Average error		_____

Name _____ Section _____ Date _____

Data Sheet: Older Adults

Subject(s) #3 Age: _____ years

Begin with this column:

12-second pre-KR 3-second post-KR			3-second pre-KR 12-second post-KR		
Direct to move	Degrees or cm moved	Error	Direct to move	Degrees or cm moved	Error
80° or 60 cm	_____	XXX	80° or 60 cm	_____	XXX
60° or 45 cm	_____	_____	60° or 45 cm	_____	_____
40° or 30 cm	_____	_____	40° or 30 cm	_____	_____
60° or 45 cm	_____	_____	60° or 45 cm	_____	_____
40° or 30 cm	_____	_____	40° or 30 cm	_____	_____
80° or 60 cm	_____	_____	80° or 60 cm	_____	_____
80° or 60 cm	_____	_____	80° or 60 cm	_____	_____
40° or 30 cm	_____	_____	40° or 30 cm	_____	_____
60° or 45 cm	_____	_____	60° or 45 cm	_____	_____
80° or 60 cm	_____	_____	80° or 60 cm	_____	_____
Total error		_____	Total error		_____
Average error		_____	Average error		_____

Subject(s) #4 Age: _____ years

12-second pre-KR
 3-second post-KR

Direct to move	Degrees or cm moved	Error
80° or 60 cm	_____	XXX
60° or 45 cm	_____	_____
40° or 30 cm	_____	_____
60° or 45 cm	_____	_____
40° or 30 cm	_____	_____
80° or 60 cm	_____	_____
80° or 60 cm	_____	_____
40° or 30 cm	_____	_____
60° or 45 cm	_____	_____
80° or 60 cm	_____	_____
Total error		_____
Average error		_____

Begin with this column:

 3-second pre-KR
12-second post-KR

Direct to move	Degrees or cm moved	Error
80° or 60 cm	_____	XXX
60° or 45 cm	_____	_____
40° or 30 cm	_____	_____
60° or 45 cm	_____	_____
40° or 30 cm	_____	_____
80° or 60 cm	_____	_____
80° or 60 cm	_____	_____
40° or 30 cm	_____	_____
60° or 45 cm	_____	_____
80° or 60 cm	_____	_____
Total error		_____
Average error		_____

Name _____   Section _____   Date _____

Data Sheet: Seven-Year-Olds

Subject(s) #5 Age: _____ years

Begin with this column:

| 12-second pre-KR | | | 3-second pre-KR | | |
| 3-second post-KR | | | 12-second post-KR | | |

Direct to move	Degrees or cm moved	Error	Direct to move	Degrees or cm moved	Error
80° or 60 cm	_____	XXX	80° or 60 cm	_____	XXX
60° or 45 cm	_____	_____	60° or 45 cm	_____	_____
40° or 30 cm	_____	_____	40° or 30 cm	_____	_____
60° or 45 cm	_____	_____	60° or 45 cm	_____	_____
40° or 30 cm	_____	_____	40° or 30 cm	_____	_____
80° or 60 cm	_____	_____	80° or 60 cm	_____	_____
80° or 60 cm	_____	_____	80° or 60 cm	_____	_____
40° or 30 cm	_____	_____	40° or 30 cm	_____	_____
60° or 45 cm	_____	_____	60° or 45 cm	_____	_____
80° or 60 cm	_____	_____	80° or 60 cm	_____	_____
Total error		_____	Total error		_____
Average error		_____	Average error		_____

Subject(s) #6 Age: _____ years

12-second pre-KR
 3-second post-KR

Begin with this column:
 3-second pre-KR
12-second post-KR

Direct to move	Degrees or cm moved	Error	Direct to move	Degrees or cm moved	Error
80° or 60 cm	_____	XXX	80° or 60 cm	_____	XXX
60° or 45 cm	_____	_____	60° or 45 cm	_____	_____
40° or 30 cm	_____	_____	40° or 30 cm	_____	_____
60° or 45 cm	_____	_____	60° or 45 cm	_____	_____
40° or 30 cm	_____	_____	40° or 30 cm	_____	_____
80° or 60 cm	_____	_____	80° or 60 cm	_____	_____
80° or 60 cm	_____	_____	80° or 60 cm	_____	_____
40° or 30 cm	_____	_____	40° or 30 cm	_____	_____
60° or 45 cm	_____	_____	60° or 45 cm	_____	_____
80° or 60 cm	_____	_____	80° or 60 cm	_____	_____
Total error		_____	Total error		_____
Average error		_____	Average error		_____

Class Data Sheet

Partners	Seven-year-olds 3 s post-KR	12 s post-KR	Class 3 s post-KR	12 s post-KR	Older adults 3 s post-KR	12 s post-KR
1						
2						
3						
4						
5						
6						
7						
8						
9						
10						
11						
12						
13						
14						
15						
16						
17						
18						
19						
20						
21						
22						
23						
24						
Total						
Average						

MEMORY PROCESSING SPEED SCORES

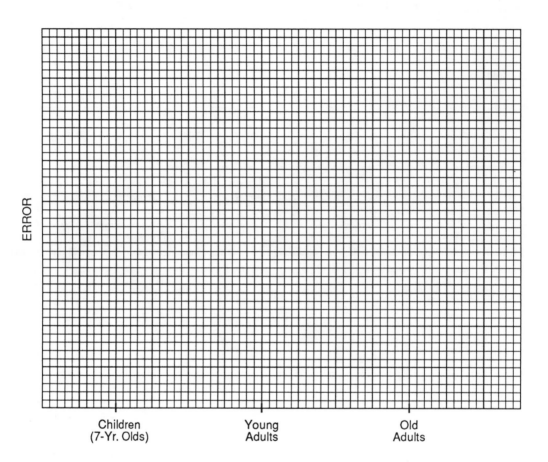

Name _____ Section _____ Date _____

Discussion Questions

1. Look at the graph. In each age group, did the length of the post-KR interval make a difference in performance? How?

2. Was there a difference among the age groups in the effect of varying the post-KR interval? If so, what was it? How did your graphed results indicate this to be the case?

3. If you observed a difference in performance over age due to varying the post-KR interval, to what do you attribute it?

(Cont.)

4. Did the results obtained by your class agree with what you expected from your readings in the textbook? If so, how? If not, speculate as to the reason.

5. After completing this experiment, how important do you feel KR is to motor performance? How did you reach this conclusion?

20

Examining Gender Role Stereotyping

Most of us are so used to the advertising and marketing messages impinging upon us daily that we neglect to question the assumptions underlying them. Recall from the discussion in chapter 9 of your textbook that toys are a facet of the socialization process. The manner in which toys are marketed to children both reflects societal attitudes and tends to maintain them. This is particularly true with regard to gender roles. Manufacturers find it advantageous to market their products along sex-typed strategies. This laboratory exercise will prompt you to examine toy marketing strategies and to decide whether these strategies socialize children into traditional gender roles.

Objectives
- To examine the packaging of toys for evidence of gender role stereotyping.
- To examine television commercials for evidence of gender role stereotyping.

Format   Independent work

Textbook Readings   "Stereotypical Behavior" on pages 265 and 266 and "Social Situations" on pages 269-271

Procedure
1. Visit a local toy store or toy section in a department store. Evaluate 20 different children's toys and how they are packaged. On the data sheet provided, enter each toy's name, its category (sedentary game, construction toy, etc.), the key word or phrase used by the manufacturer to market the toy ("just like mom's"), and whether boys or girls are pictured on the package.

2. Watch two children's programs on television. Choose a time slot popular for children's viewing rather than family viewing. Observe the commercials during and immediately following each program. Using the data sheet provided, record the name of every toy advertised, the type, the key marketing terms used, and whether boys or girls are pictured in the commercial.

Name _____ **Section** _____ **Date** _____

LABORATORY 20: EXAMINING TOY MARKETING STRATEGIES
Data Sheet: Toy Store Visit

Name of toy	Toy category[a]	Key marketing phrase	Children pictured (age, sex)

[a]Examples: construction/building set, sedentary game, make-believe domestic role (e.g., kitchen set), make-believe action career (e.g., soldier), educational toy/computer, sport equipment.

Data Sheet: Cartoon Show Commercials

Name of toy	Toy category[a]	Key marketing phrase	Children pictured (age, sex)

[a]Examples: construction/building set, sedentary game, make-believe domestic role (e.g., kitchen set), make-believe action career (e.g., soldier), educational toy/computer, sport equipment.

Name _____ Section _____ Date _____

Discussion Questions

1. Consider the category of toy. Do you find a tendency for girls to be shown with toys related to a domestic role or to mothering while boys are shown with toys related to action careers? On what do you base your answer? If you find this tendency, do you believe it serves a useful role? If so, what? Do you believe this influences boys and girls to choose certain careers?

2. If you examined any sport-equipment toys, were boys or girls pictured? Cite examples. Did the type of sport make a difference? How?

3. Consider the category of toy again. Was there a tendency for either sex to be associated with games or toys for sedentary play? For active play? Cite examples. What implications might these tendencies have for the skill development and physical fitness of children?

(Cont.)

4. What other differences did you observe in the way specific types of toys were marketed to sub-groups (sex, age, cultural group, etc.) of children?

5. Did you find food products marketed to children on television commercials? If so, what types of foods were advertised? Would a diet plentiful in these foods be a healthy one?

6. Based on your observations in this laboratory exercise, do you believe toys are a part of the socialization process, especially socialization into gender roles? On what findings do you base your answer?

APPENDIX

A

Head Circumference Percentiles

Appendix A
Head Circumference Percentiles
(in centimeters)

Age Yr. Mo.	Male Percentiles					Female Percentiles				
	10th	25th	50th	75th	90th	10th	25th	50th	75th	90th
Birth	32.8	33.2	34.3	35.2	36.0	32.1	33.1	33.8	34.5	35.3
0-1	35.4	36.2	36.9	38.0	38.6	34.4	35.4	36.3	37.0	37.8
0-2	37.4	38.0	38.8	39.8	40.4	36.6	37.5	38.0	38.9	39.4
0-3	38.7	39.4	40.4	41.1	41.9	38.1	38.8	39.6	40.4	40.8
0-4	40.1	40.7	41.4	42.5	43.1	39.3	39.9	40.6	41.4	41.8
0-5	40.8	41.8	42.4	43.4	44.1	40.0	40.8	41.5	42.3	42.9
0-6	41.9	42.8	43.5	44.3	45.0	40.9	41.7	42.4	43.3	44.0
0-9	43.9	44.8	45.3	46.3	47.1	42.5	43.6	44.1	45.3	45.8
1-0	45.0	45.7	46.6	47.2	48.1	43.9	44.8	45.4	46.5	47.4
1-6	46.8	47.4	48.2	49.0	49.7	45.1	46.0	47.0	47.9	48.8
2-0	47.6	48.2	49.1	49.9	50.7	46.4	47.1	48.1	49.0	49.8
2-6	48.3	48.9	49.7	50.5	51.2	47.0	47.8	48.6	49.7	50.5
3-0	48.8	49.5	50.2	50.8	51.9	47.4	48.4	49.3	50.2	51.1
3-6	49.2	49.8	50.5	51.4	52.1	47.8	48.6	49.6	50.8	51.6
4-0	49.5	50.1	50.8	51.6	52.2	48.2	49.1	50.2	51.2	52.0
4-6	49.7	50.4	51.2	52.0	52.7	48.6	49.4	50.5	51.5	52.3
5-0	50.0	50.7	51.4	52.3	53.1	48.8	49.7	50.8	51.8	52.6
5-6	50.4	51.1	51.8	52.7	53.4	49.1	49.9	51.0	52.0	52.8
6-0	50.6	51.2	51.9	52.8	53.6	49.2	50.2	51.2	52.2	53.0
6-6	50.8	51.4	52.2	53.1	54.0	49.5	50.4	51.6	52.4	53.3
7-0	51.1	51.6	52.3	53.2	54.0	49.8	50.7	51.8	52.5	53.5
7-6	51.4	51.8	52.5	53.4	54.3	49.9	50.8	51.6	52.8	53.5
8-0	51.4	52.0	52.8	53.6	54.4	50.2	51.1	52.0	53.1	54.0
8-6	51.6	52.2	52.8	53.8	54.4	50.3	51.3	52.3	53.1	53.9
9-0	51.9	52.3	53.1	54.0	54.8	50.1	51.2	52.4	53.3	54.0
9-6	51.8	52.5	53.2	54.1	54.9	50.3	51.5	52.6	53.5	54.4
10-0	52.1	52.7	53.5	54.3	55.2	50.9	51.8	52.9	54.0	54.7
10-6	52.2	52.8	53.6	54.5	55.4	50.9	52.0	53.0	54.0	54.8
11-0	52.3	53.0	53.8	54.5	55.3	51.1	52.1	53.2	54.1	54.8
11-6	52.4	53.1	53.8	54.6	55.5	51.2	52.2	53.2	54.6	55.4
12-0	52.7	53.3	54.0	54.8	56.1	51.6	52.4	53.7	54.8	55.9
12-6	52.8	53.4	54.2	54.9	55.7	51.8	52.6	53.7	54.8	55.8
13-0	52.8	53.6	54.4	55.1	55.9	52.2	52.8	53.9	54.9	56.2
13-6	53.1	54.0	54.8	55.5	56.3	52.1	52.8	53.9	55.0	56.2
14-0	53.4	54.2	54.9	55.7	56.5	52.3	53.0	54.2	55.4	56.6
14-6	53.5	54.3	55.1	55.8	56.4	52.7	53.3	54.3	55.7	56.5
15-0	53.6	54.4	55.3	56.1	57.2	52.4	53.0	54.3	55.5	56.7
15-6	53.7	54.8	55.6	56.7	57.2	53.1	53.8	55.1	55.8	56.5

(Cont.)

Head Circumferences Percentiles (Cont.)

Age Yr. Mo.	Male Percentiles					Female Percentiles				
	10th	25th	50th	75th	90th	10th	25th	50th	75th	90th
16-0	54.3	55.2	56.1	56.9	57.6	52.4	53.3	54.5	56.0	57.0
16-6	54.2	55.2	56.0	56.9	57.7	52.7	53.1	55.7	56.4	56.8
17-0	54.7	55.6	56.2	57.4	58.2	52.3	53.6	54.9	55.8	56.9
17-6	55.0	55.7	56.6	57.5	58.3	52.9	54.6	55.4	56.0	56.7
18-0	54.7	55.7	56.5	57.1	57.8	52.5	53.4	55.0	55.7	56.8
19-0	55.0	55.8	56.9	57.5	58.6	52.8	54.3	55.1	56.1	57.0
20-0	55.3	56.0	57.0	57.9	58.8	52.9	53.8	54.9	56.1	57.0
21-0	55.7	56.1	57.1	58.3	59.1	53.0	53.9	55.3	56.2	58.0
22-0	55.8	56.6	57.4	58.3	59.2	52.8	53.6	54.9	56.2	57.6
23-0	55.7	56.5	57.2	58.0	59.4	52.7	53.5	55.0	56.3	57.8
24-0	55.7	56.4	57.5	58.7	59.4	52.8	53.7	54.8	56.5	57.8
25-0	55.6	56.3	57.4	58.6	59.7	52.8	53.9	54.9	56.2	57.8

Note. The data are from *Human Growth and Development* (p. 130-131) by R.W. McCammon, 1970, Springfield, Illinois: Charles C Thomas. Copyright 1970 by Charles C Thomas. Adapted by permission.

APPENDIX

B

Observation Checklists

Name _____ **Section** _____ **Date** _____

OBSERVATION CHECKLIST: *Running*

Observation number	1	2	3	4	5	6	7
Runner's name							
Runner's age							
Date							
Observation type[a]							
Component							
Leg action							
Pre-run							
Step 1. Minimal flight							
Step 2. Crossover swing							
Step 3. Direct projection							
Arm action							
Step 1. Middle guard							
Step 2. Bilateral arm swing							
Step 3. Oblique arm swing							
Step 4. Opposition, sagittal							
Summary profile							
Leg							
Arm							

[a]Codes for observation type: D = direct; P = photographs; F = film; V = video; s = slow motion.

Name _____ Section _____ Date _____

OBSERVATION CHECKLIST: *Jumping*

Observation number	1	2	3	4	5	6	7
Jumper's name							
Jumper's age							
Date							
Observation type[a]							
Component							
Takeoff							
Leg							
Step 1. Asymmetrical							
Step 2. Symmetrical, bent							
Step 3. Symmetrical, full extension							
Trunk							
Step 1. Less than 30°, Neck hyperextended							
Step 2. Neck flexed/aligned							
Step 3. 30°, Neck flexed							
Step 4. 30°, Neck aligned							
Arm							
Step 1. Opposition							
Step 2. Winging							
Step 3. Guard							
Step 4. Arms flex							
Step 5. Arms flex, overhead							

[a]Codes for observation type: D = direct; P = photographs; F = film; V = video; s = slow motion.

(Cont.)

OBSERVATION CHECKLIST: Jumping (Cont.)

Observation number	1	2	3	4	5	6	7
Component							
Flight/landing							
Leg							
Step 1. One-foot landing							
Step 2. Asymmetrical, two-foot landing							
Step 3. Hip, knees flex together							
Step 4. Knees, then hips, flex							
Trunk							
Step 1. Less than 30°							
Step 2. 30°, Hyperextended							
Step 3. 30°, Flexes							
Arm							
Step 1. Opposition							
Step 2. Winging							
Step 3. Guard/windmill							
Step 4. Reach forward							
Summary profile							
Takeoff							
Leg							
Trunk							
Arm							
Flight/landing							
Leg							
Trunk							
Arm							

ᵃCodes for observation type: D = direct; P = photographs; F = film; V = video; s = slow motion.

Name _____ **Section** _____ **Date** _____

OBSERVATION CHECKLIST: *Hopping*

Observation number	1	2	3	4	5	6	7
Hopper's name							
Hopper's age							
Date							
Observation type[a]							
Component							
Leg action							
Step 1. Momentary flight							
Step 2. Fall and catch; swing leg inactive							
Step 3. Projected takeoff; swing leg assists							
Step 4. Projection delay; swing leg leads							
Arm action							
Step 1. Bilateral inactive							
Step 2. Bilateral reactive							
Step 3. Bilateral assist							
Step 4. Semiopposition							
Step 5. Opposing assist							
Summary profile							
Leg							
Arm							

Note. From *Developing Children—Their Changing Movement* (p. 54) by M.A. Roberton and L.E. Halverson, 1984, Philadelphia, PA: Lea & Febiger. Copyright 1984 by Lea & Febiger. Adapted by permission.

[a]Codes for observation type: D = direct; P = photographs; F = film; V = video; s = slow motion.

Name _____ Section _____ Date _____

OBSERVATION CHECKLIST: *Throwing*

Observation number	1	2	3	4	5	6	7
Thrower's name							
Thrower's age							
Date							
Observation type[a]							
Component							
Foot action							
Step 1. No step							
Step 2. Homolateral							
Step 3. Contralateral, short							
Step 4. Contralateral, long							
Trunk action							
Step 1. None/forward-back							
Step 2. Block/upper trunk only							
Step 3. Differentiated rotation							
Arm Action: backswing							
Step 1. No backswing							
Step 2. Elbow and humeral flexion							
Step 3. Circular, upward							
Step 4. Circular, downward							
Arm action: humerus							
Step 1. Humerus oblique							
Step 2. Humerus aligned, independent							
Step 3. Humerus lags							
Arm action: forearm							
Step 1. No lag							
Step 2. Forearm lag							
Step 3. Delayed lag							

[a]Codes for observation type: D = direct; P = photographs; F = film; V = video; s = slow motion.

(Cont.)

OBSERVATION CHECKLIST: Throwing (Cont.)

Observation number	1	2	3	4	5	6	7
Summary profile							
Foot							
Trunk							
Backswing							
Humerus							
Forearm							

ªCodes for observation type: D = direct; P = photographs; F = film; V = video; s = slow motion.

Name _____ Section _____ Date _____

OBSERVATION CHECKLIST: *Striking*

Observation number	1	2	3	4	5	6	7
Striker's name							
Striker's age							
Date							
Observation type[a]							
Component							
Racquet/bat action							
Step 1. Chop							
Step 2. Arm swing only							
Step 3. Racquet Lag							
Step 4. Delayed Lag							
Humerus action							
Step 1. Humerus oblique							
Step 2. Aligned, independent							
Step 3. Humerus lags							
Trunk action							
Step 1. None/forward-back							
Step 2. Block/upper trunk							
Step 3. Differentiated rotation							
Foot action							
Step 1. No step							
Step 2. Homolateral							
Step 3. Contralateral, short							
Step 4. Contralateral, long							
Summary profile							
Racquet							
Humerus							
Trunk							
Foot							

[a]Codes for observation type: D = direct; P = photographs; F = film; V = video; s = slow motion.

Name _____ Section _____ Date _____

OBSERVATION CHECKLIST: *Catching*

Observation number	1	2	3	4	5	6	7
Catcher's name							
Catcher's age							
Date							
Observation type[a]							
Component							
Arm action							
Step 1. Little response							
Step 2. Hugging							
Step 3. Scooping							
Step 4. Arms give							
Hand action							
Step 1. Palms up/down							
Step 2. Palms inward							
Step 3. Hands adjustable							
Body action							
Step 1. No adjustment							
Step 2. Premature adjustment							
Step 3. Delayed adjustment							
Summary profile							
Arm							
Hand							
Body							

[a]Codes for observation type: D = direct; P = photographs; F = film; V = video; s = slow motion.

8594